MAGAZINE'S

Nutrition for Peak Performance

**Eat and Drink for Maximum Energy
On the Road and Off**

EDITED BY ED PAVELKA

RODALE

Bicycling is a registered trademark of Rodale Inc.

Printed in the United States of America on acid-free ∞, recycled paper ♻

Cover Designer: Susan P. Eugster
Cover Photographer: Mitch Mandel/Rodale Images

Library of Congress Cataloging-in-Publication Data

    Bicycling magazine's nutrition for peak performance : eat and drink for maximum energy on the road and off / edited by Ed Pavelka.
       p. cm.
    Includes index.
    ISBN 1–57954–252–2   paperback
    1. Cyclists—Nutrition.   I. Title: Nutrition for peak performance.
II. Pavelka, Ed.   III. Bicycling.
TX361.C94 B535   2000
613.2'0247966—dc21   00–031090

Distributed to the book trade by St. Martin's Press

2   4   6   8   10   9   7   5   3   1   paperback

Visit us on the Web at www.rodalesportsandfitness.com,
or call us toll-free at (800) 848-4735.

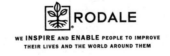

WE INSPIRE AND ENABLE PEOPLE TO IMPROVE
THEIR LIVES AND THE WORLD AROUND THEM

Notice

The information in this book is meant to supplement, not replace, proper road cycling and mountain biking training. Like any sport involving speed, equipment, balance, and environmental factors, cycling poses some inherent risk. The editors and publisher advise readers to take full responsibility for their safety and know their limits. Before practicing the skills described in this book, be sure that your equipment is well-maintained, and do not take risks beyond your experience, aptitude, training, and comfort level.

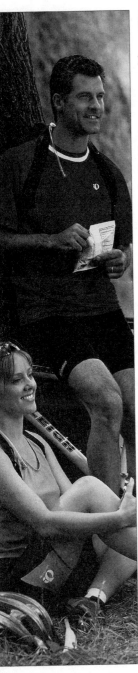

Contents

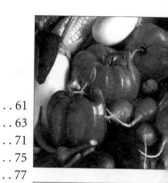

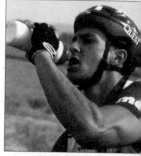

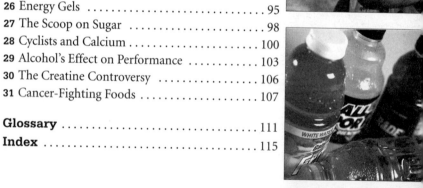

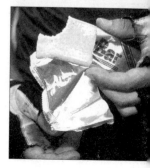

Introduction

I admit it: I don't know much about nutrition. Good cyclists are supposed to study and understand the right way to eat and drink. I manage to get by with just enough knowledge to avoid blowing off the top of my head during rides. But I wasn't always so ignorant.

A couple of decades ago, in college, I decided that road-racing bikes were irresistibly cool. In order to justify having one, I had to become a road racer. Obviously. I knew that having trick equipment is what really counts in a race. If you had skinnier tires and a lighter bike than the next guy, you would beat his pants off.

My preseason training consisted of riding "really fast" for many miles (up to 3), then stopping to pant. I got my $110 10-speed ready for the season by trading some fool my steel clincher wheels for his tubulars, complete with patched sew-up tires. I traded the padded saddle for a rock-hard nylon jobby that was ounces lighter. Best of all, having access to a machine shop, I drilled that poor bike's frame and components in places to lighten the bike even more.

The first event of the year was a 25-mile time trial. I was worried about my ability to ride the whole distance, but I had a secret edge: nutrition.

I had just seen (note that this does not mean "read carefully, absorbing the deeper meaning") an article about carbohydrate loading for distance rides in *Bicycling* magazine. With the rapidly scanned carbo article and all the drilling in my dropouts, I would really stick it to those guys with the big legs and worn-out jerseys. I got up early on the morning of the time trial and broke out a box of pancake mix. I'd never actually made pancakes, but after a few false starts, they gleamed darkly—and smoked slightly—on my plate. I poured on the syrup (lots of carbos), crammed in the whole mess, and washed it down with double-strength orange drink.

The cyclists met at the local bike shop before riding out to the course. This so-called warmup was long—at least 4 miles—and I had a hard time keeping up. I was feeling, well, loaded. I began to worry. I still had 25 miles ahead of me.

When it was my time to motor through the time trial, I sprinted off and rode incredibly fast—for about 5 minutes. Then I started feeling, shall we say, poorly. I fought against burning muscles and failing will, praying that the carbos would load up my muscles with energy soon. Very soon. By the time I got to the turnaround, 12.5 miles out—farther than I had ridden that year, incidentally—I was crawling along in a low gear, breathing like a locomotive, sweating buckets, turning several shades of green.

As I banked into the U-turn—right in front of the hundreds of gorgeous female onlookers that always came out to cheer for the local time trial—the carbos came home to roost. My turn became a death spiral, and I fell onto my side, twitching helplessly. Ra-a-a-alph! A vitreous cone of whole wheat with lots and lots of syrup hit the pavement, a monument to nutritional philosophy gone horribly wrong.

Eventually, I got to my wobbly feet and oozed back onto my oh-so-trick bicycle. A few miles down the road, as the cooling breeze dried my sweat, I began to feel better. Soon, I was skimming along at a fairly respectable speed. Not only did I finish, but I placed second from the last, beating a 72-year-old man. I owe it all to carbo *un*loading for my amazing finish.

That experience put me off one-shot dietary experiments forever. I knew I'd ride better if I dedicated some time to understanding the nuances of cycling nutrition, but where, I wondered, could I get all of the essential info in one handy place?

John Olsen
Contributing Editor
Bicycling and *Mountain Bike* Magazines

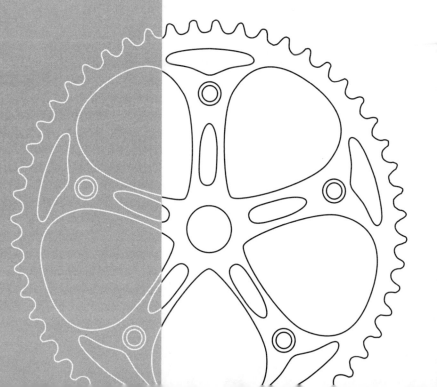

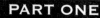

PART ONE

Elemental Eating

1
Essentials of Great Nutrition

This book explores many facets of sound nutrition for cyclists. Before getting into the specifics, here's an overview of essential concepts and core advice. This will be helpful if you've become confused by conflicting information. In fact, if you're not feeling uncertain about what to eat and drink for peak performance, it's probably because you haven't been trying to figure it out. After all, cyclists are regularly bombarded with claims (sometimes contradictory) that certain foods or diets will help them live longer, lose weight, look younger, and, of course, ride better.

If you're tired of feeling perplexed—and perhaps bouncing from one food fad to another, only to learn the hard way that radical eating plans, magic ingredients, and expensive supplements don't work—this chapter is for you. It lays the foundation for what you need to know about eating for good health and better cycling.

Fuel Number One: Carbohydrate

If you had a plate of pasta for every article written about carbohydrate, you could start your own Italian restaurant. There's a good reason, however, why sports nutritionists hype carbo: It's your best fuel.

Essentially, carbohydrate is sugar. Simple carbohydrate is a single or double sugar molecule—usually glucose, fructose, galactose, sucrose, or lactose. These are found in nutritious foods (fruits, for instance) as well as less healthful fare such as candy. Complex carbohydrate is a long chain of simple sugars and is often called a starch. Potatoes and pasta are good examples.

When you eat carbo, it's broken down and converted to blood glucose, the body's main fuel and the only type that can feed the brain. Glucose that is not immediately used for energy is stored in the muscles and liver as glycogen and is used later for fuel. If these storage spots are full, the glucose is converted to fat.

Carbohydrate is a better cycling fuel than protein or fat. Although stored protein can be converted to energy when glucose and glycogen become depleted, the process is inefficient. Stored fat can also be a fuel source, but it can't be converted to energy in the absence of glucose.

This is why you need carbohydrate. Not only does a diet that's high in fat and protein carry more calories and adverse health effects, it does a poorer job of providing energy for cycling.

During and immediately after a hard effort, simple and complex carbo is equally effective as fuel. But in your general diet, it's best to emphasize the complex type, which promotes significantly greater glycogen synthesis and offers vitamins, minerals, and fiber along with the energy.

Overall, nutritionists recommend that at least 60 percent of your calories come from carbohydrate. For cyclists and other aerobic athletes, 65 percent is better. Food packages list carbo content as a percentage of daily calories, making this fairly simple to track. To help, here's a formula that enables you to estimate the number of carbo grams you need to account for 65 percent of your diet.

First, determine your total calorie requirement by multiplying your weight by 15. To this number, add 10 calories (for men) or 8 calories (for women) for each minute of cycling you do a day. The total is roughly the number of daily calories you need to maintain your weight. (To lose weight, consume 500 fewer calories each day. You'll lose at a safe rate of 1 pound per week.)

For example, a 150-pound man who does a 1-hour training ride would figure as follows: 150 × 15 = 2,250 calories + 600 calories (60 minutes × 10 calories) = 2,850 total calories. For this rider, 65 percent of total calories amounts to about 1,850. This is the number of carbo calories he should eat daily. Because carbo has 4 calories per gram, he can divide 1,850 by 4 to determine that he needs about 460 grams of carbo a day. (2,850 total calories × 0.65 = 1,852.5 carbo calories ÷ 4 = 463 grams of carbohydrate.)

Beyond the math, the point is that you should increase your intake of whole-grain breads, fat-free dairy products, cereals, pasta, rice, potatoes, vegetables, fruits, and juices. At the same time, keep your total daily calorie consumption at the right level by decreasing your intake of fat and protein as found in meat, cheese, whole dairy products, and snack foods.

Endurance Eating

No matter how well-trained you are, your endurance is limited by one thing: the depletion of stored glycogen. When this happens, you become light-headed, dizzy, and fatigued. In cycling, it's called bonking. Fortunately, it isn't inevitable. There are ways to increase glycogen stores and prolong performance.

The best way is through training. Well-conditioned muscles can store 20 to 50 percent more glycogen than untrained ones. To take advantage of this expanded capacity, you need to eat plenty of carbo calories every day. Successive days of low intake can lead to a condition called training glycogen depletion, characterized by fatigue and lackluster performance.

For several days before an important event, pack your muscles with glycogen by reducing your riding and increasing your intake of carbohydrate to as much as 75 percent of total calories. By making more glycogen available to your muscles—and using less—you'll top off your tank for the big ride. If you have trouble consuming enough food to get all the carbohydrate you need, try a concentrated sports drink known as a carbo loader, which can supply more than 200 grams of carbohydrate per serving.

Drink for Energy

Even the world's strongest cyclist would run out of gas if he didn't refuel while riding. The reason is simple. Early in a ride, almost all of your energy comes from stored muscle glycogen. But as your glycogen levels decline, you rely more on blood glucose for fuel. To continue riding, you need to keep these sugar levels high.

One way to do this is with a sports drink. If a drink contains too much carbohydrate, however, it bogs down in the stomach and takes too long to reach the bloodstream, resulting in dehydration and possibly nausea. The most effective drinks contain just enough carbohydrate (5 to 7 percent) to empty into the bloodstream quickly, extending performance without interfering with hydration.

Some cyclists can drink fruit juice (perhaps diluted with water) or use commercial drinks with high (up to 25 percent) carbo concentrations without problems. The benefit is a bigger dose of energy per bottle. When preparing a drink, you may want to try different concentrations to find the strongest one that causes no problems. Of course, experiment during training rides, not in important events.

To be effective, a sports drink should deliver 40 to 60 grams of carbohydrate per hour. Check the ingredients and consider avoiding products that contain fructose. This is a slow-absorbing sugar that causes stomach distress in some riders. Look instead for sucrose, glucose, or glucose polymers. The last consists of several glucose molecules linked together. This chain is absorbed quickly as if it were a single molecule, but it breaks up in the bloodstream to give you the benefit of several glucose molecules instead of just one.

For rides lasting much beyond 2½ hours, you'll also want solid food. There are numerous commercial energy bars to choose from, plus good high-carbo foods such as bagels, bananas, or dried fruit. Unlike drinks, these choices do not enhance hydration. So drink plenty of water with them.

Fuel Number Two: Fat

Next to carbohydrate, fat is your body's best fuel. It's particularly useful on long, steady rides when intensity is low. But don't assume that this gives you license to eat all the ice cream and french fries you want.

True, body fat is important for storing vitamins and providing insulation. But in excess, it's one of the biggest health risks imaginable. It increases susceptibility to heart disease, high blood pressure, certain cancers, and diabetes.

Most people have plenty of stored fat, and in fact, many have too much. While people can store only limited amounts of glycogen, they can stockpile unlimited fat. Remember, though, that fat can be burned only in the presence of glucose. For these reasons, what people need is more carbohydrate, not more fat.

Any kind of food can turn into body fat if you eat too much. But not surprisingly,the most likely source for body fat is dietary fat. Compared with protein and carbohydrate, dietary fat has more than twice as many calories (9 per gram rather than 4), and it appears to be stored more readily.

For optimal health and performance, nutritionists recommend that you derive no more than 30 percent of your total calories from fat, and no more than 10 percent from the saturated fats found primarily in animal products. The remainder should be the unsaturated form that comes from vegetable oils, nuts, and grains.

One way to ensure a low fat intake is to check nutrition labels and select foods with less than 3 grams of fat per 100 calories. If this information isn't plainly listed, you can calculate the fat percentage this way.

Look on the label for the grams of fat per serving. Multiply this number by 9, then divide the result by the calories per serving. The result is the percentage of calories from fat. For example, 1 ounce of processed cheese spread has 80 calories and 6 grams of fat. So, 6 grams of fat × 9 calories per gram of fat = 54 fat calories. Fifty-four ÷ 80 (total calories) = 67.5 percent calories from fat. (To figure a food's percentage of calories from carbohydrate or protein, multiply the number of grams by 4 instead of 9. Then divide by total calories.)

Trim fat from your diet by reducing your intake of animal foods. When you do consume them, select lean cuts of meat, skinless poultry, and fat-free dairy products. Also, cut down on butter and margarine, salad dressings, and hydrogenated and tropical oils (prevalent in many baked goods).

Interestingly, the fitter you are, the better you burn fat. A well-trained body is capable of delivering more oxygen into the muscles, thus increasing the rate of fat metabolism and sparing some glycogen stores.

Fuel Number Three: Protein

Cyclists do require more protein than sedentary people. But this doesn't mean you have to increase your protein intake. In fact, you're probably already getting more than you need.

One reason cyclists need extra protein is for fuel. Once muscles have depleted their primary energy source (carbohydrate), they begin using protein as well as fat. According to researcher Michael J. Zackin, Ph.D., of the University of Massachusetts Medical School, "Protein can be a small but significant source of energy—about 5 to 10 percent of total energy needs. Protein calories become increasingly important in carbohydrate-depleted states. If you train more than an hour a day and begin to deplete glycogen stores, you become increasingly dependent on body protein for energy."

Though results vary widely, Dr. Zackin says cycling may raise your protein requirements 20 to 90 percent beyond U.S. Recommended Dietary Allowances. The Recommended Dietary Allowance, or RDA, is 0.363 gram of protein per pound of body weight. For a 150-pound man, this is about 54 grams per day. For a 120-pound woman, it's about 43 grams. Add the 20 to 90 percent and the male cyclist's daily protein need rises to 65 to 103 grams, the woman's to 52 to 82 grams.

That may seem like a lot, but most active people are already at these levels or beyond. This was illustrated in a study of eight highly trained women cyclists. Though their diets fell short of recommended values for several nutrients, their protein intakes were 145 percent of the RDA. High protein levels simply aren't hard to reach. For instance, 3 ounces of meat, fish, or poultry contain 21 grams. A cup of beans has 14 grams, 3 tablespoons of peanut butter have 12 grams, and a cup of fat-free milk contains 9 grams. All of this adds up quickly. In fact, the average American consumes 100 grams of protein per day.

So unless you're a strict vegetarian or chronic dieter, you probably don't need to increase your protein intake. Instead, worry about where your protein comes from. The best sources are low in fat and include a healthy dose of complex carbohydrate. Muscles are built by work, not extra protein, and work is best fueled by carbohydrate.

Some low-fat, high-protein choices include whole grains, beans, vegetables, fish, skinless poultry, soy products, lean cuts of meat, and fat-free dairy products. Even vegetarians can get plenty of high-quality protein with a varied diet combining grains, legumes, nuts, seeds, vegetables, dairy products, and eggs.

Overall, nutritionists say that about 15 percent of your diet should be protein calories. But don't sweat it—this is one nutrition goal you'll reach without even trying.

Amino Acid Supplements

Protein helps build muscle tissue, and protein is nothing more than a strand of amino acids. This is why many athletes take amino acid supplements. The theory is that by augmenting your diet with pills or powders, you'll build muscle. In reality, though, this doesn't work.

Because most people get more than enough protein in their diets, few have amino acid deficiencies. Any excess, whether it comes from food or heavily hyped supplements, is burned inefficiently as a fuel or turned into fat, not muscle. In great excess, amino acid supplements can even lead to dehydration, calcium loss, and liver or kidney damage.

Even if extra amino acids were beneficial, the best way to get them isn't through pills or powders. Like vitamins, the best way is through food. In fact, on an average day, most people ingest tens of thousands of milligrams of amino acids.

"Most supplements provide 200 to 500 mg of amino acids per pill, while an ounce of chicken supplies 7,000 mg," says Ellen Coleman, R.D., coauthor of *The Ultimate Sports Nutrition Handbook*. She notes that chicken also supplies other essential nutrients. In addition, getting the same amount of amino acids from supplements as you would from an ounce of chicken might cost as much as 20 times more.

Vitamins and Minerals

It's much the same for vitamin and mineral supplements. As with amino acids, you almost certainly get everything you need if you're eating a well-balanced diet. According to Coleman, "As a cyclist, your vitamin and mineral requirements are no greater than those of a sedentary person. Remember, vitamins do not provide a direct source of energy. Their only purpose is to help people with nutritional deficiencies stemming from poor diets."

No research has found that taking supplements improves performance in well-nourished cyclists. On the other hand, some substances can actually accumulate in the body to dangerous levels if taken in large quantities. Too much niacin, for example, can cause rashes, nausea, and diarrhea. It can also interfere with the body's ability to burn fat for fuel. This forces you to use glycogen at a faster rate, which makes you fatigue quicker during a ride.

At about a dime per dose, a daily multivitamin/mineral supplement is often viewed as cheap insurance, so go ahead if you want to be sure all bases are covered. But if you're feeling tired or your performance is slipping, don't expect supplements to help. The cause is probably overtraining or eating too little carbohydrate, not the lack of some vitamin. As Coleman notes, "When people feel better after taking vitamin and mineral supplements, it's usually due to the strength of their belief that they'll help—the placebo effect."

Diets and Weight Loss

Looking for long-term weight loss that will improve your cycling performance? Part Three contains an in-depth discussion of this subject. For now, a quick piece of advice: Trash the crash diets. Sure, some weight (mostly water and lean body mass) may come off quickly, but it usually returns just as fast.

To take off fat—and keep it off—you must make two permanent (and almost painless) lifestyle commitments. The first is easy: Exercise. Make time to ride. Don't let yourself go more than 2 days without it. Studies show that you can stay trim with as little as 3 hours of exercise per week.

The second commitment is harder: Cut calories. The best way isn't to eat less but to reduce your fat intake. In the average American diet, nearly 40 percent of all calories come from fat. Trim this to 20 to 30 percent and you're almost guaranteed to lose weight.

Remember that fat is twice as calorie-dense as protein or carbohydrate. So as long as your foods aren't fatty, you can eat plenty and still keep your calorie intake relatively low. For example, in a study at Cornell University, subjects were put on either a 40-percent or 15-percent fat diet and allowed to eat all they wanted. Both groups ate similar amounts, but those in the 15-percent group averaged 700 fewer daily calories.

2
Good Health, Good Cycling

It's no coincidence. The same foods that play a role in the prevention of heart disease, stroke, and cancer also enhance cycling. In fact, a high-carbohydrate, low-fat diet does it all. It fortifies you for consecutive days of training while increasing your odds of a long, healthy life. What's not so well-known is exactly how such a diet is best used to boost riding performance.

For example, you need to eat to have energy for cycling, but you should avoid eating less than 2 hours before a ride begins. This ensures that your stomach will be empty enough that you won't become nauseated. Actually, a preride meal isn't a major source of energy for short outings. Your real fuel comes from the energy stores you've built with your daily diet. (For long rides, it's different. You must eat and drink while riding in order to keep up with your energy requirements.)

The best way to build and replenish your energy stores is with carbohydrate. Both the complex and simple types supply your body with glycogen—the most efficient muscle fuel for cycling. But complex carbo (fruit, vegetables, beans, cereals, whole-grain breads) also offers several specific health advantages. For instance, the soluble fiber in oats, beans, and fruit reduces blood cholesterol. The insoluble fiber in wheat bran, whole-grain products, and vegetables (particularly their skins) main-

The Best Complex Carbo Sources

FOOD	PORTION	CARBOHYDRATE (G)	CAL	CAL FROM CARBOHYDRATE (%)
Fruit juice	1 c	30	120	100
Dried fruit (raisins, apricots)	⅓ c	40	160	100
Corn on the cob	1 ear	29	120	95
Banana	1 large	27	115	94
Baked potato	1 large	51	220	93
Rice, white cooked	1 c	50	223	90
Dry cereal	1 c	25	110	90
Spaghetti, cooked	1 c	34	160	85
Corn grits, cooked	1 c	31	146	85
Kashi, cooked	1 c	38	177	84
Wheat bulgur, cooked	1 c	47	227	83
English muffin	1	30	150	80
Rice cakes	5	40	200	80
Pita bread	1 pocket	21	106	79
Popcorn, plain	4 c	18	92	78
Bread sticks	4	30	154	78
Pancakes (4 in.)	3	51	260	78
Pretzels, low-salt	2 oz	43	222	77
Bagel	1	31	160	77
Kidney beans, canned	1 c	35	186	75
Bread	2 slices	30	160	75

tains healthy bowels. And fruits and vegetables rich in vitamin C and beta-carotene protect against certain types of cancer. For these reasons as well as your performance needs, about half of your daily caloric intake should be made up of complex carbo.

Conversely, simple carbo should constitute less than 10 percent of your daily calories. Be careful about eating sweets such as cake and candy before riding. As will be discussed in chapter 3, the hormone insulin, which is secreted by the pancreas to counteract the influx of sugar, may lower blood sugar levels too much for some riders. This can cause weakness and light-headedness while riding.

The Skinny on Fat and Protein

Just as there are two types of carbohydrate, there are two kinds of fat: saturated and unsaturated. Saturated fat, such as butter, is solid at room temperature and is derived mainly from animals (with the exception of palm and coconut oils, which are highly saturated vegetable fats). Unsaturated fat, such as corn oil, is liquid at room temperature and is derived mainly from plants.

A high-fat diet, particularly when the fat is saturated, increases blood cholesterol—a major risk factor for heart disease. It also increases the risk of certain types of cancer. Both the American Heart Association and the National Cancer Institute recommend that no more than 30 percent of your calories come from fat. Yet many Americans take in much more.

For a cyclist, excess fat can be especially disastrous. You need to maintain your muscle glycogen stores by fueling up on complex carbo, and this can't be done on a high-fat diet. Your body's slow digestion of fat (compared to carbo) can also make you sluggish. If you ride 1 hour a day, about 60 percent of your calories should be derived from carbohydrate. If you ride several hours a day, make it 70 percent. This will ensure that your glycogen stores are full.

Your body uses protein chiefly for tissue growth and repair. Your daily calorie intake should include 10 to 15 percent from protein. Most people meet this requirement with ease. If you consume more protein than you need, it'll either be used for energy or turned into body fat. Excess protein can also contribute to dehydration because your kidneys need more water to process it. Dehydration can impair cycling performance, even on rides as short as an hour.

Ideal Diets

To achieve a balanced diet for good health and to ensure that you have the energy needed for cycling while keeping your calories low, try the following recommended menus for low- and high-mileage riding. If you find that you're losing weight, increase your caloric intake.

If You Ride an Hour or Less a Day

Men should eat 2,000 calories. In this example, 57 percent of calories come from carbohydrate, 29 percent from fat, and 14 percent from protein.
Breakfast: ⅓ cup bran cereal; 1 cup low-fat milk; one banana; one slice raisin toast; ½ cup grapefruit juice

Lunch: Tuna melt sandwich made with two slices whole-wheat bread, 3 ounces tuna mixed with celery, green onion, 1 teaspoon mayonnaise, 1 ounce Cheddar cheese, and 1 tomato slice; several carrot and celery sticks; 1 cup apple juice; 1 cup low-fat yogurt with 1 cup raspberries

Dinner: Stir-fry made with 2 teaspoons peanut oil, 4 ounces skinned chicken, and 1½ cups vegetables; 1½ cups brown rice; one orange

Snack: 1 cup low-fat milk and one medium blueberry muffin

Women should eat 1,500 calories. This menu derives 56 percent of total calories from carbohydrate, 27 percent from fat, and 17 percent from protein.

Breakfast: 1 cup Cream of Wheat with 2 tablespoons raisins; ½ cup orange juice

Lunch: Sandwich made with ½ whole grain pita bread, ⅓ cup seasoned garbanzo beans, lettuce, tomato slice, and onion; ½ cup cooked broccoli; ½ mango; 1 cup low-fat milk

Dinner: 4 ounces lean beef; baked potato with 2 teaspoons margarine; ½ cup spinach salad with 1 tablespoon French dressing; yogurt shake made with 1 cup low-fat yogurt, ½ banana, and ¼ cup strawberries

If You Ride More Than an Hour a Day

Men should eat 3,000 calories, of which 69 percent come from carbohydrate, 18 percent from fat, and 13 percent from protein

Breakfast: 1 cup orange juice; 1 cup oatmeal with sliced banana; 1 cup low-fat milk; 2 slices wheat toast with 2 teaspoons margarine

Lunch: Sandwich made with two slices rye bread, 3 ounces turkey, 1 ounce mozzarella cheese, lettuce, one tomato slice, and 1 teaspoon mayonnaise; 1 cup apple juice; one orange; 1 cup lemon sherbet

Snack: Eight graham crackers; 1 cup low-fat milk; one apple

Dinner: 2 cups spaghetti with ⅔ cup tomato sauce, mushrooms, and 2 tablespoons Parmesan cheese; four slices French bread with 2 teaspoons margarine; ½ cup broccoli; ½ cup ice cream with ¾ cup strawberries

Snack: 6 cups air-popped popcorn

Women should eat 2,500 calories, of which 70 percent come from carbohydrate, 16 percent from fat, and 14 percent from protein

Breakfast: 1 cup grapefruit juice; 1 cup Cream of Wheat with ½ cup blueberries; 1 cup low-fat milk; 2 slices wheat toast with 2 teaspoons margarine

Lunch: Sandwich made with two slices wheat bread, 3 ounces lean beef, 1 ounce Monterey Jack cheese, lettuce, one tomato slice, and ½ teaspoon mustard; 1 cup grape juice; one orange; 1 cup orange sherbet

Snack: Four graham crackers; 1 cup low-fat milk; one apple

Dinner: 2 cups spaghetti with ⅔ cup tomato sauce, mushrooms, and 2 tablespoons Parmesan cheese; two slices French bread (easy on the margarine); ½ cup broccoli; ½ cup ice cream with ¾ cup strawberries

Snack: 3 cups air-popped popcorn

3
How Food Becomes Energy

When you reach into your jersey for a banana during a ride, that piece of fruit begins a journey more fascinating and magical than even the greatest bicycle tour. By the end of its trip, your banana—or sandwich or energy bar or whatever you ate—is transformed into energy, the key to completing your ride.

Along the way, several interesting changes occur. Edward Coyle, Ph.D., a cyclist and leading carbohydrate researcher as the director of the Human Performance Laboratory at the University of Texas at Austin, chronicles these alterations. He lives in a fascinating world of questions: What should you eat before a ride? How can food and drink combat fatigue? What type of riding is best for losing weight? How concentrated should a sports drink be? To what extent can food and drink extend endurance?

The answers begin with a piece of food and its three main compounds: protein, carbohydrate, and fat.

Fuel Sources

Your body breaks down the energy stored in the molecules of the food, explains Dr. Coyle. Protein is rarely used for energy, but it does play other crucial roles in your body. Carbohydrate, on the other hand, is the preferred source of energy because your body can break it down fast. Therefore, it rapidly releases the energy you need for a vigorous ride.

Dietary fat is a stored energy source, either in your blood as free fatty acids, in your muscle fiber, or beneath your skin. You burn more body fat on long, slow rides, which is why easy efforts are often recommended for losing weight. According to Dr. Coyle, however, this logic is flawed. He contends that an hour of slow riding will burn fat, but when you eat later, the calories you consume will only replenish these fat stores. A better weight-loss approach, therefore, is to burn as many calories as you can by riding hard. In any case, no matter how you look at it, fat is the body's secondary fuel source.

When your body is forced to use fat as an energy source, you are limited to exercising at no more than 50 to 60 percent of your aerobic capacity, says Dr. Coyle. For instance, if you can normally hold a top speed of 24 mph, you won't be able to ride much faster than 15 mph for more than 5 to 10 minutes. Fat obviously is a limiting source of energy. Consider that if you're on a fairly intense ride, maintaining a heart rate of 150 to 160 beats per minute, you get only about 40 percent of your energy from fat. The rest comes from carbohydrate—your body's fuel of choice.

Glycogen Stores

As carbohydrate travels through your digestive system, it is converted into its storage form, known as glycogen. Then, it takes one of two paths. Some carbohydrate goes to the liver, where it's converted into glucose, a principal energy source of living organisms. This quickly enters the circulatory system as blood glucose. Meanwhile, other carbohydrate is stored in the muscles as muscle glycogen. This process, however, occurs at a much slower rate.

Early in a ride, you rely almost exclusively upon muscle glycogen for energy, explains Dr. Coyle. But as your muscle glycogen levels decline, you rely more on blood glucose. In just 3 hours of riding, the percentage of carbohydrate energy coming from muscle glycogen steadily declines from 100 percent to zero, while energy from blood glucose increases from zero to 100 percent.

So after a few hours of pedaling without eating, your glycogen and glucose stores will be depleted. Even if you have ample fat stores, the process through which these are converted to energy is not efficient enough to sustain your riding effort. With less fuel reaching your brain

Carbohydrate Calorie Counter

FOOD	PORTION	CAL
Cereals		
Cheerios	1¼ c	111
Corn Chex	1 c	111
Rice Chex	1⅛ c	112
Shredded Wheat with fruit	½ c	100
Wheat Chex	⅔ c	104
Cookies and Crackers		
Animal crackers	15	120
Fruit bars, raisin-filled biscuits	1	53
Gingersnaps	7	115
Graham crackers	4	120
Vanilla wafers	7	130
Fruit		
Apples		
dried	¼ c	52
fresh	1	81
Apricots, dried	¼ c	78
Banana	1	105

and muscles, you'll begin to feel dizzy and fatigued. Eventually, you'll bonk.

But what if you had been ingesting carbo-rich food and liquid during the ride? Could such feedings replenish your blood glucose stores fast enough to forestall the bonk?

At one time, the scientific consensus was no—carbohydrate feedings couldn't contribute significant energy for exercise. The thinking was that sugary drinks couldn't be used rapidly enough by the body. But Dr. Coyle and others found that this theory isn't correct. "The body can use carbohydrate during the latter stages of exercise when muscle glycogen is very low," he says. "We tested cyclists between the third and fourth hour of a ride and found that they weren't using any muscle glycogen. All their carbohydrate energy was coming from the glucose they were drinking."

Dr. Coyle has shown that if cyclists eat and drink while riding, they

FOOD	PORTION	CAL
Blueberries	1 c	82
Figs	¼ c	127
Grapes	½ c	57
Orange	1	62
Peaches, dried	¼ c	96
Pears		
dried	¼ c	118
fresh	1	98
Prunes	¼ c	96
Raisins	¼ c	109
Raspberries	1 c	61
Strawberries	1 c	45
Miscellaneous		
Bagel, plain	1	160–200
Fruit roll-up	1 (½ oz)	50
Pita bread with sliced fruit or shredded vegetables, plain or with 1 tsp low-calorie dressing	1	165

can extend their endurance, despite the fact that their muscle glycogen stores are exhausted. In one study, he had two groups of cyclists ride to exhaustion, then ingest either a placebo or carbohydrate. When they resumed riding 20 minutes later, those who ingested the carbohydrate were able to cycle 45 minutes longer.

Normally, if you start to fatigue, the end of your riding energy comes quickly. You bonk and you're done. But with steady carbohydrate feeding, you're able to grind it out despite increasing fatigue.

Correct Concentrations

After determining and demonstrating the effectiveness of carbohydrate feeding, Dr. Coyle turned to dispelling some other myths.

For instance, experts once believed that a sports drink should not contain more than 2.5 percent carbohydrate. It was thought that anything more would slow the solution's passage from the stomach to the intestines. This would have two negative effects. First, it would take longer for the body to absorb the fluid, thus inhibiting its ability to cool itself by sweating. Second, such slow emptying would cause nausea.

Dr. Coyle agrees that high concentrations of carbohydrate can slow gastric emptying, but he disagrees about the consequences. "The stomach can empty a liter of water per hour, but it can only empty 800 milliliters per hour of a 5 percent carbohydrate solution," he explains. "Statistically, this is significant. But functionally, it doesn't constitute a big difference. No one has been able to prove that the slowdown in gastric emptying makes any difference in the body's ability to cool itself."

In fact, some studies have shown the opposite. A research group at Ball State University in Muncie, Indiana, compared the effects of ingesting 5-, 6-, and 7-percent solutions during a long ride. The tests resulted in an extended performance for each rider who participated.

Meanwhile, a University of South Carolina study compared 6- and 12-percent solutions. This one was conducted at 91°F to gauge the effect on sweating. The 12-percent dose did not alter the body's ability to cool itself. It did cause some upset stomachs, however.

Indeed, nausea is the main reason extremely high concentrations are still not universally accepted. When Dr. Coyle fed cyclists a 10-percent carbohydrate solution, 10 percent of the subjects vomited. "When you start ingesting solutions that have 7 to 10 percent or more carbohydrate, it can build up in the stomach and cause gastric distress," he explains. "But it's very individual. Some people can tolerate any concentration and empty it quickly. The key is to experiment to find what's best for you."

Dr. Coyle notes that during exercise, the body can draw glucose from the blood at the rate of 1 gram per minute, or 60 grams per hour. Thus, to be effective, a sports drink should deliver between 40 and 60 grams of carbohydrate per hour. To accomplish this, you can either drink a little of a very concentrated solution or a lot of a diluted solution. Doing the latter will also help you meet your fluid replacement needs. With a 2.5-percent solution, however, you would have to drink several liters per hour, which isn't realistic.

The Unfounded Fear of Hypoglycemia

Another bit of dated logic contends that eating carbo-rich foods immediately before a ride stimulates the secretion of insulin, a hormone that actually removes glucose from the blood. When combined with exercise, this can result in a dramatic drop in blood glucose, a condition called hypoglycemia. The symptoms include cold sweat, headache, confusion, hallucinations, convulsions, and even coma. At the very least, it's said that the scarcity of glucose leads to light-headedness and lower performance. But Dr. Coyle sees it differently.

"It's overrated. Most riders never sense it," he says. "We've found that fewer than 25 percent of those who experience hypoglycemia ever have a central nervous system effect where they feel shaky or irritable. Early in a ride, it's of almost no consequence. Only one in 30 people notices the effects. Later, they'll notice the depletion of blood glucose because they're depriving their muscles of energy. At this point, they may be able to tolerate the effects of hypoglycemia, but they can't tolerate the fact that their legs lack energy."

By ingesting carbohydrate throughout the ride, Dr. Coyle continues, you're providing your muscles with extra energy, so you're able to ride longer. Then why, you might wonder, can't you just keep ingesting carbohydrate and cycle indefinitely?

"Nobody knows," says Dr. Coyle. "We've studied cyclists riding with low levels of muscle glycogen but high levels of blood glucose. Their muscles seemed to be taking in glucose adequately. But after extending the exercise for about an hour, they had a second fatigue and they stopped. Something else is going on other than carbohydrate. We just don't know what."

A study at the University of Waterloo, Ontario, has also concluded that other unknown factors, not carbohydrate availability, cause fatigue. One suspect is an electrical change within the muscles. But even if science can't as yet enable you to pedal indefinitely, you can improve your cycling performance and extend endurance by using carbohydrate correctly, especially on glycogen-depleting rides of 3 hours or more. Here are some tips for your next epic ride.

■ A few days before a long ride, "ingest 600 grams of carbohydrate per day," says Dr. Coyle. This will have your glycogen stores brimming. To achieve this, you may want to try one of the carbo-loading drinks on the market. They're designed to augment glycogen stores.

■ A few hours before a long ride: "It doesn't make much difference what you eat," says Dr. Coyle, "as long as you've eaten well the previous few days and the night before."

■ During a ride: "On any ride longer than 3 hours," says Dr. Coyle, "bring bagels, a sports drink—anything high in carbohydrate. Liquids are easier to consume and provide necessary fluid. I suggest a carbohydrate concentration between 5 and 10 percent in volumes of 200 to 400 milliliters every 15 minutes." (A typical water bottle holds 600 milliliters.)

"But don't ignore solid food," he continues. "All carbohydrate is treated the same way by your body. In fact, it's good to mix solids with fluids, especially on long rides. I work with cycling teams and provide them with all types of carbohydrate fluid alternatives during races and hard rides. But once they've been riding about 6 hours, they all say the same thing: 'I want something solid.'"

4
Dietary Hits and Misses

Most foods—even a grease-soaked, bacon-wrapped double cheeseburger with mayo and a large side of fries—have some nutritional value. Despite the obvious danger, they probably won't kill you, provided you indulge only occasionally. Conversely, the healthiest food choices can be risky if that's all you eat. (Remember fads like grapefruit- or cabbage-only diets?)

Your health depends on your whole diet, not just on whether you eat certain foods or avoid others. For day-in, day-out health, there are good choices and bad choices. Here are some of each.

Ignore These at Your Peril

1. Whole grains. These have more vitamins, minerals, and fiber than refined varieties. High-fiber diets protect against colon cancer and help regulate cholesterol levels. Include whole grains at breakfast (cereals such as Cheerios, All-Bran, Shredded Wheat, or hot oatmeal), at lunch (whole-wheat tortillas, pitas, sandwich bread), and dinner (brown or wild rice, whole-wheat pasta). Your goal is six or more servings per day—not hard to accomplish if you down a little at each meal.

2. Whole fruits. Whole fruits provide more fiber and more variety, and are more satisfying to your hunger pangs than juice is. Top-rated choices are the red and orange types (cantaloupes, oranges, mangos, apricots, red grapefruits, strawberries). In many cases, their color comes from naturally occurring pigments that are potent antioxidants (thought to be good for cancer prevention). Of the two to four servings of fruit you should eat each day, make at least two of them whole fruits.

3. Low-fat dairy products. For adults up to age 50, the National Academy of Sciences recommends 1,000 milligrams of calcium daily and for those over 50, 1,200 milligrams . If you're not getting at least three servings of dairy products, chances are, you're not meeting these recommendations. Calorie for calorie, fat-free milk is a great nutritional package. One 8-ounce glass provides 30 percent of your calcium needs and more than 10 percent of the recommendations for protein, potassium, vitamins A, B_{12}, D, and more—in only 80 calories. Try it straight up, on cereal, in lattes, or in things you would usually mix with water (such as hot chocolate or hot cereal). Low-fat yogurt is also great as a snack—or blend milk, yogurt, and fruit into a smoothie.

4. Deep-green vegetables. Vegetables in this group fill four of the five top slots in a list of most healthful vegetables compiled by the Center for Science in the Public Interest, based in Washington, D.C. They're a nutritional gold mine, providing necessities like carotenoids, vitamin C, folate, and potassium—as well as that healthful old standby, fiber. Good choices include broccoli, romaine lettuce, brussels sprouts, spinach, and green peppers. You need at least three veggies each day—and one should be deep green.

5. Lean protein. Some cyclists put all their efforts into choosing high-carbohydrate, low-fat foods. But you shouldn't reduce quality protein too much. Athletes need more protein than sofa spuds, and getting too little can lead to loss of muscle mass as well as increased susceptibility to illness. Lean cuts of meat, fish, and poultry are concentrated

What's In There?

To find out more about the things you eat, check out the Food and Nutrition Information Center Web site (www.nal.usda.gov/fnic). It has extensive information on food composition and safety. In addition, it has links to other valuable nutrition resources.

sources of high-quality protein and other valuable nutrients such as iron, zinc, and vitamin B$_{12}$. You don't need a lot—one or two portions a day, the size of the palm of your hand. Other good sources include dried peas and beans, tofu, or low-fat cottage cheese.

Avoid These like Glass in the Road

1. Raw eggs. Many raw eggs contain salmonella, truly nasty bacteria that cause nausea, vomiting, diarrhea, and in some cases, death. This little bug, also found in undercooked chicken and meat, causes almost 60 percent of the cases of food-borne illness. Unrefrigerated foods (for example, at picnics) pose a particular risk. Here's the rule to go by: Keep hot foods hot and cold foods cold until you eat them.

2. Hard margarine. "Stick" margarine is usually made with vegetable oils, but hydrogenation (used to make liquid oil into solid margarine) results in trans fatty acids. From the heart-health perspective, these are as harmful as saturated fat. To cut down, use a soft (tub) margarine, or even better, buy a nonhydrogenated margarine with no trans fat.

3. Soda. The typical can of soda has almost 10 teaspoons of sugar and few, if any, redeeming features (although it does provide water). If you brush and floss your teeth, the sugar won't be a problem. In fact, your muscles can't tell if glucose comes from sugar or whole grains. But for the same calories, you'll do better by drinking fruit juice or milk. If it's just fluid you're after, go for water.

4. Full-fat sour cream. Baked potatoes are a great food choice—but not if they're smothered in sour cream, which is high in fat and contributes relatively little to taste. So moisten that spud with juice from your veggies or meat, or add a dollop of low-fat yogurt.

5. Double cheeseburger wrapped in bacon. Yes, the hamburger contains protein and the cheese provides some calcium. Some versions even come with lettuce and tomato. But these nutritional plusses are packaged with more than 1,000 calories, a whopping 60 percent of which are from fat, especially if you don't say "hold the mayo." Go for a turkey on rye at the deli instead.

5
Beware of the Zone

Sometimes, it seems that nutrition advice is hooked to a gigantic pendulum. If you don't like the recommendations today, just wait and they'll change. The carbohydrate pendulum began swinging for athletes in 1939 when Swedish scientists found that men on a normal diet (about 50 percent carbo) could exercise for 2 to 3 hours compared to only 1 hour on a very low carbo diet (less than 5 percent of daily calories). What's more, they could exercise for up to 4 hours on a 90 percent carbo diet.

Further work in the late 1960s confirmed these differences and demonstrated that a high-carbohydrate diet produces greater muscle glycogen stores. In the 1980s, athletes subsisted on pasta, bagels, and bananas, living in mortal fear that even a trace of fat might pass their lips. Then, in the 1990s, the Zone, or 40/30/30 diet, came on the scene.

Instead of recommending approximately 60 percent of calories from carbohydrate, this diet suggests only 40 percent, with a whopping 30 percent from protein (compared to the usual recommendation of 10 to 15 percent). It also recommends the typical 30 percent of calories from fat.

Here's a look at carbohydrate's role in the cyclist's diet from three important perspectives: overall health, weight management, and cycling performance.

Carbo's Role

In terms of overall health, several decades of research have led the U.S. Surgeon General and numerous other health authorities to recommend a higher-carbohydrate, lower-fat diet that's rich in fruits, vegetables, and whole grains. Such a diet is associated with lower risks of major chronic diseases including hypertension, atherosclerosis (clogging of the arteries), and certain cancers. At this point, there's no evidence to suggest that this advice should be ignored.

As for weight management, proponents of the 40/30/30 diet claim that high carbohydrate intakes cause obesity. According to the theory, too much carbohydrate stimulates the pancreas to release excessive amounts of insulin (the hormone that clears glucose from the blood-

How Much Protein Is Enough?

Studies have shown that athletes need more protein than your typical couch potato. Suggested intakes for athletes are 1.2 to 1.5 grams of protein per kilogram (2.2 pounds) of body weight, compared to the Recommended Dietary Allowance (RDA) of 0.8 gram per kilogram. But athletes also consume more calories, and this helps provide them with enough protein.

The amount recommended in the popular 40/30/30, or Zone diet, is excessive. For instance, imagine you're a 132-pound (60-kilogram) cyclist who requires 3,000 calories per day to fuel training and daily activities. (Insert your own weight to personalize these recommendations. Your weight in pounds divided by 2.2 equals your weight in kilograms.) Using the commonly suggested 1.2 to 1.5 grams of protein per kilogram, you'd need 75 to 90 grams daily. This represents 10 to 12 percent of 3,000 calories. (One gram of protein has 4 calories.) This could be readily met by a normal diet, which provides 70 to 100 grams of protein per day.

To reach 30 percent protein (the amount called for in the Zone diet), however, you'd need to consume a massive 224 grams. Here's what you'd need to eat each day.

1 cup cottage cheese	28 g
1 can (3 oz) tuna fish	22 g
3 glasses low-fat milk	24 g
8 oz lean beef	66 g
1 cup kidney beans	13 g
¼ cup peanut butter	32 g
1 chicken breast	27 g
3 egg whites	12 g
Total	224 g

This amount of protein is excessive by any standard. Potential risks include strain on the kidneys and bone loss. (Excreting excess protein increases urinary calcium loss, potentially compromising bone health.) The latter may be of particular concern to cyclists because cycling isn't a weight-bearing activity, and weight-bearing activities are necessary to promote bone strength.

In contrast, you could meet the normal diet's protein requirement of between 70 and 100 grams if you consumed 1 cup of cottage cheese (28 grams), 1 chicken breast (27 grams), 2 glasses of milk (16 grams), and 1 cup of kidney beans (13 grams). This totals 84 grams, which is well within the range of a normal diet. The milk and cottage cheese provide calcium and, compared to the load of food required to reach 224 grams of protein, you'll have much more room for glycogen-producing carbohydrate.

stream). Over time, the body becomes resistant to insulin, causing the pancreas to secrete even larger quantities. High levels of insulin stimulate fat synthesis and prevent the fat stored in body cells from being used.

This almost makes sense. Unfortunately, it's a case of putting the cart before the horse. Obesity, not high carbohydrate intake, causes insulin resistance. Over time, too many calories from any source increase body fat stores, which in turn lead to insulin resistance. Insulin sensitivity can be restored by weight loss. A 1997 British study showed that obese subjects who shed weight maintained their weight loss better on higher-carbohydrate diets. Several other studies confirm that, other things being equal, fewer calories are consumed on these diets. There's an important qualifier here, though: Low-fat doesn't necessarily mean low calories, so don't inhale a whole box of low-fat cookies rather than the two or three you might have had otherwise.

What is most interesting is what a low-carbo diet does to cycling performance. Over the years, literally hundreds of studies have been conducted on the effects of nutrients consumed before, during, and after exercise. Many factors affect the results: the level at which the subjects are trained, the intensity and duration of the exercise, and even the gender of the subjects. But there's little debate that carbo before and during moderate-intensity endurance exercise is beneficial and that carbo shortly after exercise helps restore muscle glycogen.

Controversy exists, however, around the question, "How much carbo is needed on a day-to-day basis?" The medical literature contains numerous studies showing improved performance with carbohydrate intakes of 60 to 70 percent of calories (compared to 50 percent or less), yet a few show no difference—or even improved performance with lower carbohydrate intakes. Most experts agree, though, that the evidence continues to favor carbohydrate.

It is possible that some athletes—those who overdo carbohydrate and nearly exclude protein—could benefit from slightly higher protein intakes, although not at the 30 percent level. But for increased endurance as well as general health, moderation and balance in your diet are important—regardless of nutrition's pendulum motion.

6

Special Needs for Women

Women cyclists have special needs both on the bike and in the kitchen. Unfortunately, like the general population, many riders seem to think that fat and calories are the two most important aspects of nutrition. Actually, a bigger boost on the bike will come from satisfying your body's specific nutritional requirements, especially in terms of iron and calcium intake. The simple dietary changes described in this chapter will improve your cycling, strengthen your bones, and help you reach your optimum weight.

Consider More Iron

Iron directly affects your cycling performance. It's an integral component of hemoglobin, the compound that carries oxygen to working muscles. Too little oxygen being taken up and used by muscles is the major factor limiting endurance performance in cycling and other activities. If your iron deficiency progresses to anemia, where hemoglobin levels drop to dangerous levels, even a low-effort, leisurely ride can feel exhausting.

During the childbearing years, a typical woman's Recommended Dietary Allowance (RDA) of iron is 15 milligrams. That's 50 percent more than what men need. The main reason is that women lose iron each month in their menstrual flow. So it's no surprise that women with heavy periods are at greater risk for deficiency than women with a lighter menstrual flow.

To get more iron, consider eating more red meat. It's probably the best dietary source because it contains heme iron, which is absorbed more efficiently than iron from plant foods. If red meat doesn't appeal to you, good nonanimal sources include fortified breakfast cereals and dried beans and legumes. Also eat foods that are rich in vitamin C (orange juice, green peppers, potatoes) because they increase iron absorption from plant foods. When cooking, use cast-iron cookware, which naturally boosts the iron content of your meals, especially when you're making foods that contain vitamin C, such as tomato sauce or hash brown potatoes.

The amount of iron in multivitamin and mineral supplements is safe. But therapeutic doses (30 milligrams per day or more) should be used only with a physician's advice for treatment of anemia because this much iron can interfere with absorption of other minerals.

Boost Calcium

Getting enough calcium is crucial for female cyclists. Intense forces such as those produced by running increase bone strength, but the smooth motion of pedaling does not stimulate a similar benefit. While many athletes have higher bone density measurements than normally active people, cyclists and swimmers do not.

The latest calcium RDAs are the same for men and women: 1,000 milligrams per day up to age 50, and 1,200 milligrams per day thereafter. But a U.S. Department of Agriculture national survey found that women average only 635 milligrams daily, compared to 879 milligrams for men. So the calcium gap is greater for women—a big concern because women's risk for osteoporosis is higher than men's. Your diet can do a lot to fix the deficit if you use these guidelines.

Get three a day. Consume three servings daily of low-fat dairy products. In addition, choose foods that are calcium-fortified.

Use a supplement. Experts recommend food sources over pills, but if you can't meet the requirement through diet, a supplement will help.

Drink your milk. Moo juice (or a fortified soy beverage) is one of the few food sources of vitamin D, which works with calcium to build bone. So if you don't drink milk, and especially if you're over 50, consider supplemental vitamin D.

Put down the saltshaker. Go easy on sodium and avoid excessive protein. Each can contribute to calcium loss.

Cross-train. Weightlifting, running, tennis, basketball, and aerobics are all good ways to promote bone strength. The key is that these activities make your skeleton bear your body weight (as opposed to when you're sitting on a bike seat).

Consider hormones. Talk to your doctor about hormone-replacement therapy if your periods are irregular or absent. Decreased exposure to reproductive hormones can lead to rapid bone loss.

Emphasize Fitness Instead of Weight

"If I had one wish as a nutritionist," says Susan I. Barr, Ph.D., a long-distance cyclist, nutritionist, and professor at the University of British Columbia in Vancouver, Canada, "it would be for women athletes to spend less time obsessing about calories and weight and more time enjoying food and activity. Weight simply isn't the best measure of health in active adults. Research at the Cooper Clinic in Texas shows that physically fit but overweight people have fewer health risks than their unfit but normal or underweight counterparts."

But if you still want to shed a few pounds without unreasonably restricting your diet and jeopardizing good health, here's how: Increase your cycling intensity. Forget what you may have heard about low-intensity exercise being best for burning fat. The harder you go, the more total calories you use per minute of riding.

Modify your diet with fresh fruits and veggies; low-fat or fat-free dairy products; and lean fish, poultry, or meat. You'll notice that these are the same foods that provide calcium, iron, and other essential minerals. After losing 5 pounds, let your body get used to the new weight. Don't attempt to lose more until your strength returns to normal.

7
10 Ways to Improve Your Diet Today

Here you are, determined to eat better and get fitter. Again. Chances are, you've tried several times in the past. Usually, such resolutions don't last because they contain words like *never* (as in, "I will never eat junk food again"), or they're much too general. Despite your good intentions, you set yourself up for failure even before you start.

Instead, be specific and realistic. For example: "I will cut some fat from my diet by snacking on pretzels instead of chips." Rather than try to change everything at once, take small but effective steps that address one key aspect of your diet at a time.

With this in mind, here are some very doable suggestions that will help you eat better and ride better. Begin using them today and enjoy the results.

1. Drink enough on every ride. Studies done more than 50 years ago prove that maintaining hydration substantially improves endurance and helps prevent cramps. Unfortunately, too many cyclists take their bottles for a ride instead of drinking the contents. Drinking on the bike is a learned skill, and needs practice. A trick: Set the countdown timer on your watch to go off every 12 minutes, and drink when it beeps. Your goal should be to finish every ride weighing what you did at the start, which usually means at least one bottle of fluid per hour.

2. Follow the "five-a-day" rule. When it comes to fruits and veggies, you should be eating at least five items each day. These food groups help prevent cancer, heart disease, and constipation while providing energy-rich carbohydrate. What a deal! They're convenient, too—keep bags of scrubbed baby carrots, prewashed salad fixings, or fruit and vegetable juice in the fridge. To start, strive for five servings at least 5 days a week.

3. Eat breakfast. Believe it or not, people who eat breakfast extend their life spans and weigh less, according to a study conducted in California. And eating before a morning ride extends your endurance. A good breakfast doesn't have to take much time, either. Try whole-grain cereal with fruit and milk, or a bagel with peanut butter and jam. Even a commercial meal replacement drink is a good start. If you're an avowed no-breakfast person, give it a try for 2 weeks. You'll see the benefits even if you're not trying to lose weight. Studies show that breakfast skippers tend to eat more total calories during the day.

4. Bone up on calcium. Bone health is maintained by the combination of calcium and weight-bearing exercise. Because bike riding isn't weight-bearing, cyclists need to pay close attention to calcium intake and add cross-training to their routines. How much calcium is enough? At least 1,000 milligrams per day for people under 50 years old, or 1,200 milligrams per day for those over 50. This means three high-quality calcium servings daily, such as milk, yogurt, cheese, or calcium-fortified products like certain cereals and fruit juices (check labels). Order a café latte, have hot chocolate made with milk at bedtime, or snack on low-fat ice cream to boost your calcium intake. Men: Remember that bone health isn't just a women's issue. You can get osteoporosis, too, so follow these calcium guidelines.

5. Eat on longer rides. You'll ride stronger if you take in some energy during the first hour and continue to do so throughout the ride. Remember that the form can be solid (energy bars, cookies, fruit), liquid (sports drinks) or carbo gels. With gels or bars, make sure that their wrappers can be opened easily while you're riding. Or, open the bars at home and rewrap them in wax paper before tucking them in your jersey.

Depending on your body size, aim for 30 to 60 grams of carbohydrate per hour. (A typical energy bar contains 40 grams. Check the label.)

6. Cut the fat. Some of us still eat more fat than we need for good health and good cycling. In a Danish study, men undergoing an 8-week training program made greater performance gains on high-carbohydrate diets than on diets high in fat. Cutting fat also leaves room to increase your intake of performance-enhancing carbo. (Active adults should get about 25 to 30 percent of total daily calories from fat.) The key: Find specific, realistic changes that work for you. For instance, have your bagel with jam instead of cream cheese, or use mustard instead of mayonnaise on your sandwich.

7. Emphasize whole grains. Many cyclists follow the nutritional gospel of high-carbohydrate intake, but they don't emphasize the right kind. Your muscles may not be able to tell the difference between squishy white bread and crunchy whole-grain varieties (both provide fuel for pedaling), but there's a big difference in their nutritional value. Whole grains win hands down, with more fiber, vitamins, minerals, and phytochemicals (for cancer prevention). So think "whole grain" and "brown" when it comes to foods such as cereal, bagels, pitas, rice, and pasta.

8. Pop a pill. Taking a multivitamin/mineral supplement each morning probably won't make you a better cyclist, and it definitely won't fix a poor diet. But if you're already eating well, it will make sure that you're getting enough folic acid, for example, which is important in preventing heart disease and birth defects. Despite a good diet, you may have an insufficient intake of certain nutrients, making a daily supplement cheap insurance.

9. Escape your dietary routine. Do you eat the same foods day in and day out? Even though bagels, peanut butter, bananas, pasta, and fruit juices are healthful foods, they don't make a healthful diet if they're all you eat. Make a resolution to try something you've never eaten before at least once each month—or better yet, once each week.

10. Stay positive. Any self-improvement resolution, no matter how well-crafted, is doomed to failure if you become a slave to it. Remember, eating for health is more than individual nutrients and fat phobia. A healthful diet in an active lifestyle such as cycling has room for an occasional rich piece of chocolate cake. Look at it as a reward, not a failure.

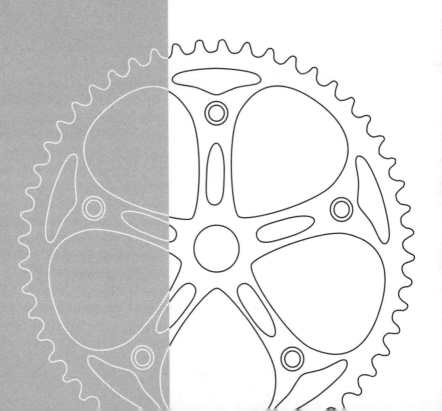

PART TWO

Food
on the Move

8
Meals on Wheels

This chapter is by Davis Phinney, the winningest road racer in U.S. cycling history. Before retiring from competition, Phinney was a member of the 1984 Olympic cycling team and went on to win two stages of the Tour de France. Today, he runs the Carpenter/Phinney Cycling Camps in Boulder, Colorado, with his wife, Connie Carpenter, arguably the greatest woman cyclist in U.S. history.

In the spring of 1985, I rode my first Milan–San Remo classic, at 186 miles one of the longest races on the European professional calendar. An experienced Belgian rider gave me the inside scoop, or so I thought: Eat as much as possible in the first 60 miles so as to have plenty in reserve for later. I dutifully jammed my jersey pockets full of fruit, cookies, and the little ham and jelly sandwiches, called *panini*, that served as race food at the time.

Only 30 miles into the cold and rainy race, as I polished off my fourth panini, legendary Irish rider Sean Kelly pulled alongside and chirped in his high-pitched voice: "Hey boy, lay off the food or you won't even make the first climb." Besides blowing my psyche (I instantly pictured myself zeppelin-size), I soon learned that overeating is not the way to go. And thinking back, I have to laugh. Ham?

Today, the market overflows with energy bars, gels, and drinks—sport-specific energy replacement. This is a windfall to cyclists, but the choices can be confusing. What and how should you eat and drink, and when?

Tank up. Water loss through both sweating and exhalation (breathing out) will hurt your performance quicker than anything else if deficits aren't made up. Especially in warm weather, make sure that you drink at least 16 ounces of fluid (primarily water) per hour. And depending on your weight and fitness, you might need more. On longer rides, it is difficult and taxing to carry large amounts of liquid. Knowing where you can restock en route is key. As a pro rider, I often went for hours without drinking due to inattention—not a healthy habit. In hard races, where the focus switch had to be flipped on full-time, I learned that I had to drink continuously but in small doses. Backpack-type hydration systems (such as those from Blackburn, CamelBak, or Ultimate Direction) make long rides possible without water stops. And you're more likely to drink with the nozzle conveniently by your mouth as a reminder.

Fuel up. Glycogen (the gas for your engine) needs to be replenished, too, but this is a little trickier than with fluids. My rule of thumb is that higher levels of intensity require simpler forms of carbohydrate (sports drinks, gels, and fruits). It is only at lower heart rates and on longer rides that more complex foods, like those ham and jelly sandwiches, can be better utilized as fuel sources.

Are you looking for a fuel that covers the wide variety of effort you face on hilly or fast group rides? Try energy bars. In the 1986 Tour de France, my 7-Eleven teammates and I showed up with a new food that a Californian named Brian Maxwell had concocted in his kitchen. It was the first time PowerBars were introduced to the European cycling scene. In a few short weeks, the eating traditions that had ruled pro racing for years were reevaluated. Energy bars now fill the pockets of most pros. During long races, I often consumed three or four bars along with some fruit and drink, and that was all I needed.

Determine your needs. Everyone is different, so see what works for you. As a general guideline, try for a steady intake of 200 to 300 calories during each hour of riding (this comes to half an energy bar every 30 minutes). Again, fitness and ride conditions are the determining factors. Remember that calorie requirements can be met by sports drinks as well as food. In cold temperatures, you'll eat more solid food than in hot temperatures, when your appetite is suppressed and fluid intake is even more vital. There are plenty of sports drinks to choose from. Find a flavor you like so that you won't mind drinking a lot. In hot weather, it's a good idea to dilute the solution or it'll taste too sweet and syrupy.

Battle the bonk. Sometimes you just bonk—run so low on glycogen that you begin feeling weak and dizzy. To prevent this emergency from stopping you cold, always carry some packets of energy gel (Gu, Clif-Shot, PowerGel). These rapidly enter your system and are ideal pickups from GDCW syndrome (glycogen depleted, completely wasted). Carry some money for refueling at convenience stores when that notion to explore makes a ride last a lot longer than your food supply.

Picnic out of your pockets. In the old days, jerseys were made with chest pockets. Riders would pack sugar cubes in them for bonk protection. Fashions change, and jersey pockets have moved to the back, but they're still the place to carry everything from fuel to spare clothes. You can stick a gel pack under the leg of your shorts along the thigh for easy access. Store an emergency energy bar and a $10 bill in your seatbag.

Learn how to eat while riding. Opening and eating energy bars and even drinking from a bottle, particularly when riding near other people, is scary at first. When I began racing, I used to get nervous inside a fast-moving, tightly packed group. Trying to fuel up while looking cool and controlled was tough for this rookie when surrounded by pros, but with practice it became easier.

Don't try to ride with no hands while eating in a group. Crashing yourself and others is a major faux pas, and the legacy will follow you forever. Keep food in the left or right of your jersey's three rear pockets so that it's easier to reach. Drink from the down tube–mounted bottle until it's empty, then switch it with the full seat-tube bottle. In pacelines, eat and drink only when you are at the very back. On hilly courses, wait until the pace eases or you're over a climb before eating anything solid. It's hard to choke down an energy bar when your heart rate is maxed out and you're puffing like a locomotive.

Pack gourmet. There is something to be said for going retro. If you want to show up at your next club ride looking like an elegant Italian pro (at least food-wise) from the 1970s, here's how the European teams prepare race food: Panini on white bread are cut into bite-size squares after removing the crust (which is hard to digest). The filling usually consists of ham and cheese or cream cheese and jelly, but nearly anything goes. Wrap them in foil (but it's more authentic to use waxed paper) for protection from mud, dust, and perspiration. Fruit (apples, bananas, figs, kiwi, grapes, melon) is cut into small pieces and either put in plastic baggies or wrapped in foil. All of these things can easily be squished, so pack gently. No doubt you'll have the most stylish snacks of your group.

9
Fuel for the Long Haul

Have a century or epic trail ride coming up? You may need to rethink your diet. If you're eating more protein and fat than carbohydrate or saving your carbo-loading for the night before the ego-challenge, don't blame your body if it fails you en route.

For most cyclists, optimal carbohydrate intake is essential, though you'll also hear from advocates of high-protein, low-carbo diets. Chris Jensen, M.S., R.D., nutritionist for Team Shaklee, says he'd like to see more scientific data before he would recommend sacrificing carbohydrate for protein. Like Jensen, many traditional exercise physiologists and elite riders are still carbo-committed.

For optimal energy, sports nutritionists recommend getting 60 to 65 percent of calories from carbohydrate, 10 to 15 percent from protein, and up to 30 percent from fat. This nutritional formula provides all essential nutrients while reducing risk for heart disease, hypertension, diabetes, obesity, and many cancers. New evidence reveals that a high-carbo diet also helps prevent certain eye diseases, impotence, degenerative disc problems, and hearing loss.

Energy Sources

During exercise, energy comes from the carbohydrate stored in the muscles, liver, and bloodstream. At low intensities, fat is primarily burned for fuel. Unless you're riding at a snail's pace, you're burning some carbo, too, says Craig Horswill, Ph.D., research scientist at the Gatorade Exercise Physiology Laboratory. But as your engine revs higher, beyond 70 percent of your max VO_2 (your maximum aerobic ability), carbohydrate supplies the bulk of energy. Carbo's downside: Your body can store only about 1,400 to 1,800 calories, whereas it has almost unlimited fat stores to use as fuel. Each time you ride, you use some of your limited carbohydrate. Pedal at high intensity for 90 minutes, or more slowly for longer periods, and you may bonk—feel dizzy, weak, and unable to keep riding at your current pace because you're out of fuel.

An active cyclist should eat 3 to 4.5 grams of carbohydrate per day for each pound of body weight—about 450 to 675 grams of carbo for a 150-pound male. (Check food labels for carbo content.) That's a lot of carbohydrate, so try to get at least the minimum amount. Eat even more if you're gearing up for a multiday endurance ride.

Strategic Eating

Pay attention to diet details the week before an important long-distance event, such as a 100-mile ride. Contrary to popular belief, successful carbo-loading for a century isn't a preride pasta party. Instead, store more glycogen in your muscles during the 3 or 4 days before the big event by tapering exercise and eating primarily carbohydrate. Several studies of trained cyclists who loaded properly showed that they could ride farther, and often faster, than those who did not top off their glycogen stores. Studies also showed that up to 50 percent of trained "unloaded" cyclists couldn't complete a 3-hour ride at 70 percent of their max VO_2, whereas virtually all cyclists who carbo-loaded could.

Before the ride. Because everyone tolerates food before events differently, eat something familiar 2 to 4 hours before the start. Eat before training rides to get used to having something in your stomach. Don't skip breakfast. Pre-exercise, high-carbo meals—liquids, solids, or sweets—have consistently proven to enhance performance.

During the ride. Consume 30 to 60 grams of carbohydrate per hour while riding, says Dr. Horswill. That's about 16 ounces of most sports drinks. Eat energy bars, carbo gels, or your favorite pocket fuels for additional energy. Tour de France and Race Across America riders often consume 100 grams of carbohydrate per hour.

After the ride. For a few hours after a ride of 90 minutes or longer, your body can convert carbohydrate into muscle glycogen faster than normal. After this so-called glycogen window closes, the storage rate slows, and you need an entire day or more to completely restock.

This means that if you miss the window and ride again within 24 hours, you're probably doing so with only partially energized muscles. You're weaker, and you'll tire sooner. But if you use the window, you can be sure you're cycling with the optimum amount of energy in your body. Taking advantage of this window is simple. It opens anytime you participate in an aerobic sport for longer than 90 minutes. Be sure to do these things after a ride.

Refuel as soon as possible. Immediately after a ride, the window is completely open and the conversion from carbo to glycogen is quickest. In 2 hours, it closes about halfway, and the rate is cut roughly in half. During the next 2 to 4 hours, it closes to normal.

Take in enough. The optimum amount of carbo to put in your body seems to be at least 50 grams during the first 2-hour period, according to Michael Sherman, Ph.D., a professor in exercise physiology at Ohio State University in Columbus and researcher of carbo synthesis. Some scientists contend that taking up to 100 grams every 2 hours may increase the rate, but no one has proven this.

Do it with carbohydrate. The window works best with high-carbo food. A 3-day study that followed two groups of endurance runners in training showed this. Both ate at the same time during the window, but one group ate 70 percent carbo, the other 40 to 60 percent. By day three, the amount of muscle glycogen in the high-carbo group was about the same. They were recovering just about everything they lost. But the low-carbo athletes stored 75 percent less.

In terms of conversion speed, it makes no difference whether the carbo comes from liquids or solids. Liquids leave the stomach sooner, but they aren't synthesized into glycogen and stored in the muscles any faster than solid carbo.

But, says Dr. Sherman, "because by consuming liquid you're also hydrating the body, many cyclists prefer sports drinks over food for the first refueling. Many also find it easier on their stomachs right after a hard ride. Try both."

Drink to This

During cycling, your muscles produce 30 to 100 times more heat than when you're at rest. The body extinguishes this inferno primarily by increasing sweat rate. In the summer, you can lose more than 2 liters (about 67 ounces) of fluid per hour on a hot day. If you don't replace it, power output declines in about 30 minutes. A study of trained cyclists found that they could barely finish a 2-hour ride at 65 percent max VO_2 without fluids. According to *Bicycling* magazine's Fitness Advisory Board member Arnie Baker, M.D., in ultra-endurance cycling events such as the Race Across America, dehydration and saddle sores are the leading reasons cyclists drop out.

Studies by Edward Coyle, Ph.D., director of the Human Performance Laboratory at the University of Texas, reveal that cyclists who lose a quart of fluid experience a rise in heart rate of eight beats per minute, a decrease in cardiac function, and an increase in body temperature. Dehydration is also cited for increased metabolic stress on muscles and faster glycogen depletion. It wreaks havoc on your internal thermostat by decreasing bloodflow to your skin, slowing sweat rates, and increasing the time needed for fluids to be absorbed into your bloodstream. What's worse, by the time you feel thirsty, your body has already lost up to 2 percent of body weight—about a quart of fluid.

Is your mouth feeling dry just reading this? Here are several ways to beat the dehydration monster.

Drink more. Conventional wisdom calls for eight glasses of fluid daily (about 64 ounces)—but that's for nonexercising couch potatoes. Cycling wisdom calls for 1 milliliter of fluid for every calorie you burn, according to Mitch Kanter, Ph.D., director of the Gatorade Sport Science Institute. "At about 3,500 calories a day, you'll need around 3½ liters. That's almost 15 (8-ounce) glasses of fluid." He advises gauging hydration by monitoring these simple markers.

■ Do you go to the bathroom less than three times during an 8-to-10 hour workday?

■ Is your urine dark yellow and have a strong odor?

■ Do you get headaches toward the end of a long ride or shortly after?

■ Do you drink less than one water bottle per hour while riding?

■ Do you lose more than 2 pounds during rides?

If you answer yes to any of these questions, your body is heading for a drought.

Prehydrate. Drink plenty of fluids every day, but before a race, long ride, or tour, start hyperhydrating at least 24 hours in advance. Smart cyclists keep a water bottle with them all day to stay hydrated. Avoid drinks containing alcohol or caffeine because both act as mild diuretics, causing the body to excrete more water. If you have trouble meeting your calorie needs, use sports drinks, recovery drinks, or other liquid supplements. If you're weight-conscious, quaff calorie-free or low-cal options such as diluted fruit juice, mineral water, or club soda.

Set a sipping schedule. To negate fluid lost to perspiration, practice drinking strategies during training. Determine your sweat loss per hour by weighing yourself before and after rides. (Every pound lost equals 16 ounces of fluid.) Then figure how much fluid your stomach can tolerate per hour and the best drinking schedule to replace it. Dr. Kanter recommends that you set your sports watch to alert you to drink 4 to 8 ounces every 15 minutes regardless of whether you're thirsty. It takes practice to drink more than a quart per hour without intestinal discomfort. A backpack-style hydration system provides easily accessible water to help you drink more.

Rehydrate. After you've ridden for several hours, pump down fluids. What you drink makes a difference. In a study published in the

International Journal of Sports Medicine, Dr. Coyle compared the effects of drinking nearly 2 liters of water, sports drink, or diet cola in dehydrated athletes 2 hours after exercising. Results revealed that diet cola replenished 54 percent of fluid losses; water, 64 percent; and sports drinks, 69 percent.

Munch on salty snacks. Sodium makes your blood spongelike so that you absorb more water and excrete less. "Each liter of sweat saps 500 to more than 1,000 milligrams of sodium," notes Lawrence Armstrong, Ph.D., of the University of Connecticut Human Performance Lab.

Dr. Coyle suggests that athletes drink plentifully with meals and snacks because food naturally contains many times more sodium than sports drinks or energy bars.

Eat "wet" foods. About 60 percent of your daily fluid comes from the food you eat, but some foods increase hydration better than others. For instance, fruits and vegetables are great fluid sources—they're 80 to 95 percent water by weight. Eating the recommended five-plus daily servings of produce means you'll get a lot of extra water in your diet. If you're downing protein supplements, you should drink more. Dr. Kanter warns, "You'll need more water to metabolize and excrete the extra protein." He adds that fat and water don't readily mix, so many high-fat foods provide little additional water.

Use sports drinks. Most popular sports drinks contain sodium, potassium, and other electrolytes. These are recommended for exercise lasting more than 1 hour. Whenever you plan to cycle for several hours, make sure you have two bottles of your favorite. Sports drinks are also useful for shorter workouts that include high-intensity riding such as sprints and intervals.

Make sure you like the way a drink tastes so that you'll be motivated to put down lots of it. Also, cool fluids taste better and may be absorbed more rapidly than warm ones. Ed Burke, Ph.D., an exercise physiologist and a member of *Bicycling* magazine's Fitness Advisory Board, tells cyclists to carry two bottles—one frozen. As you drink down the first bottle, the frozen one melts so that the liquid is cold when you need it.

10

Beat the Bonk

You've been riding for several hours, feeling great and enjoying the scenery. But now your riding partner's chatter is beginning to irritate you. Halfway up the next hill, you go to the shift lever and discover that you're already in your lowest gear. You struggle toward the top, where your partner is waiting with a curious look on his face.

"What's this jerk looking at?" you grumble. "This is a stupid ride. I should have stayed home and mowed the lawn."

Wait a minute. What's going on here? A few minutes ago you felt great, and now you feel terrible. Why? Simply put, you've bonked.

It's a humorous word that's traditional in cycling, and that's why you've already encountered it in this book. But it's never funny when it happens. In fact, bonking is such a miserable experience that avoiding it should be a primary objective of your cycling nutrition. On any long ride, much of what you eat and when you eat it should be geared toward fending off the bonk's drastic consequences. Here is what causes it and what you can do to prevent it.

Your Energy System at Work

Bonk describes the symptoms that occur when your body's essential carbohydrate stores are depleted as a result of sustained exercise. As you ride, most of the fuel being oxidized, or burned, is consumed by your active muscles. Both fat and carbohydrate can be used for this process. Fat, stored in fatty tissue, is reduced to free fatty acids and transported by the blood to the working muscles. In contrast, carbohydrate is stored within muscles as glycogen, which is a long polymer composed of many glucose molecules. During exercise, individual molecules are removed from the polymer and used as energy.

Your vital organs also require a continuous supply of fuel. Whether at rest or during exercise, your brain and nervous system, for instance, depend upon blood glucose. The reason is that their cells don't store glycogen and can't use fat. Thus, to meet energy requirements, your blood glucose levels must be tightly regulated and maintained. This job is largely done by your liver, which contains large stores of glycogen that can be converted to glucose.

With the muscles and organs vying for glucose, extended exertion can drain the liver. When blood glucose levels become too low to meet the fuel requirements of your central nervous system, you begin feeling disoriented, tired, irritated, and generally miserable. In a word, you bonk.

Quick Remedy

Fortunately, you can cure the bonk. When your blood glucose levels fall as a result of liver glycogen depletion, you can replenish them by eating or drinking something rich in carbohydrate. This is quickly digested into simple sugars that enter the bloodstream and are transported to the liver, muscles, and other organs.

Even better, you can avoid bonking in the first place by frequently eating or drinking small amounts of carbohydrate while riding. This enables your stomach to continuously add glucose to the blood. In turn, this greatly reduces the drain on your liver's valuable glycogen stores. The trick is to begin eating or drinking about 15 minutes into a long ride and continue to do so every 10 to 15 minutes thereafter.

Of course, eating on short rides isn't necessary. But the definition of "short" and "long" depends on your fitness. For beginners, an hour-long ride is very long. For veterans, 2 hours might be short. A good preventive measure is to never leave home without your favorite energy food or sports drink—just in case.

Hitting the Wall

Although bonking and "hitting the wall" are often used interchangeably, there is a difference. Both problems result from fuel depletion. Unlike bonking, however, which is caused by the depletion of liver glycogen, hitting the wall stems from the depletion of muscle glycogen. Bonking is avoidable and curable. Hitting the wall can be delayed by ingesting carbohydrate. Once it happens, however, you're essentially finished for the day.

Hitting the wall is terminal because as the rate of fuel consumption rises in response to intensifying exercise, the muscles turn to their most readily available fuel—the glycogen stored inside. In fact, it's the only fuel that can support exercise at levels greater than 70 percent of your max VO_2. When you run out of muscle glycogen, you're able to exercise only at very moderate intensity. (Another reason muscle glycogen is so important is that it provides an essential intermediate product that's required to burn fat.)

As with beating the bonk, the key to avoiding the wall is maintaining a steady intake of carbohydrate. Another trick is to not waste the muscle glycogen you have. For instance, each time you accelerate rapidly or push hard on a steep hill, your body switches to an anaerobic metabolism to meet the extra energy demands. This process—which is so demanding that your body can't take in enough oxygen to sustain it—uses glycogen much less efficiently than aerobic metabolism. Therefore, on long rides, always accelerate smoothly, avoid blasting up hills, concentrate on your breathing, and don't be tempted into riding harder than usual.

Best Carbo Sources

In addition to sports drinks and energy bars, there are many common, less expensive sources of glycogen-producing carbohydrate. These include fig cookies, fruit bars, bananas, dried fruit, and granola bars. As with sports drinks, experiment with different solid foods. Most riders settle on a combination of solid and liquid supplements.

Whatever you select, remember to use it. It's amazing how many experienced riders bonk or hit the wall with their pockets full of food. By sipping and nibbling every 10 to 15 minutes, you'll be able to avoid the bonk. And when the ride is over, you may still have plenty of energy for mowing the lawn.

11
Countdown to a Century

After months of deliberation, you've registered for your club's annual century ride. You've signed the waiver absolving organizers of all responsibility in the event of your untimely death, and put the check in the mail. Now what?

It's time to start eating smart. Here's a pre-event nutritional countdown for a 100-mile ride, along with advice on what to eat and drink after the start of the event.

4 Weeks in Advance

Contact the organizers to find out exactly what fluids and foods will be available on the course. If you don't currently use the sports drink or some of the main food items they'll be providing, get accustomed to them by using them in training.

1 Week Before

Will carbohydrate-loading help? The answer is definitely "yes" for events as long as a century (6 to 8 hours for most recreational riders). Carbo-loading can increase your endurance by about 20 percent. To do it, gradually taper your training during the last week, ending with a rest day or an easy spin the day before the event. That way, dietary carbohy-drate can be stored as muscle glycogen rather than used as exercise fuel.

You'll need to eat more carbo than usual for the last few days of the week—up to 10 grams per kilogram (2.2 pounds) of body weight. If you gain weight, you'll know it's working, because each gram of glycogen is stored with 3 grams of water. Filling your tank with 300 to 500 grams of glycogen should produce a gain of about 5 pounds. Don't worry, it's mainly fluid, which is helpful during the event.

For a ride of 2 hours or less, a carbo-loading phase isn't essential, es-pecially if you eat a substantial pre-event meal and consume a sports drink while riding.

1 to 2 Days Before

Regardless of your event's distance, it's critical to begin well-hydrated. This doesn't mean gulping a water bottle minutes before the start. Ac-cording to the American College of Sports Medicine, based in Indi-anapolis, you should start pushing fluids at least 24 hours ahead of time. Keep a bottle close at hand all day and keep nipping at it.

The Morning of the Ride

While you were tossing and turning last night, liver glycogen was breaking down to maintain your blood glucose levels. If this glycogen isn't restored by eating a carbo-rich meal, hypoglycemia (low blood sugar) can develop during the ride and contribute to premature exhaus-tion.

In fact, eating the right pre-event meal is probably one of the most important steps you can take. It should include the following:

Breakfast of Champions

It's important to eat 1 to 4 hours before beginning a long ride. Aim for 50 grams of carbo for each hour before the start (for example, 150 grams for a meal 3 hours prior to the race). Here are some tasty breakfast suggestions.

FOOD	CARBOHYDRATE (G)
Cinnamon roll	60 plus
Bagel	50–60
Dry cereal (1½ c)	30–50
Liquid meal replacement (10 oz)	30–40
Yogurt (6 oz)	30–40
Sweetened oatmeal (¾ oz)	30–35
Banana	30
Raisins or dates (¼ c)	30
Fruit juice (1 c)	25–30

■ Foods you like and know you can tolerate when your nervous system is in overdrive. If you can't handle solid food, try meal-replacement beverages such as Ensure or Boost.

■ High-carbohydrate foods, including as much as 200 grams of carbo for meals eaten 4 hours before the event. (See "Breakfast of Champions")

■ Relatively little fat, so stomach emptying isn't delayed.

■ Fluid. If it's caffeinated, also drink an equal volume of a noncaffeinated beverage. The American College of Sports Medicine recommends about 500 milliliters (a water bottle or so) 2 hours before the event to promote hydration and allow time to excrete excess fluid.

During the Ride

During long events, it's important to start downing fluid and carbohydrate immediately. An Australian study showed that starting carbo intake right away and spreading it out over 2 hours of cycling led to better performance than consuming the same amount of carbohydrate after 90 minutes of cycling.

How much carbohydrate? At least 0.6 gram for each kilogram of body weight per hour, or about 30 to 60 grams per hour.

Liquid, solid, or gel? They all work, but solids can be difficult to eat when you're riding hard. Liquids help you meet carbohydrate and fluid needs simultaneously. One standard bottle of sports drink containing 6 to 8 percent carbohydrate provides 37 to 50 grams of carbo.

How much fluid? Ideally, enough to balance your sweat losses. But if this isn't possible, aim for 600 to 1,200 milliliters every hour (1 or 2 water bottles).

12
What's in Store?

Susan met the Grim Reaper face-to-face during a 120-mile tour on a deserted forest road in central Oregon. She'd started riding at 7 A.M. in persistent, driving rain with temperatures in the mid-40s. As she climbed, the rain turned to sleet. Despite good rain gear and layers of clothing, she couldn't remember ever feeling colder or more desperate. She began to lose contact with her arms, feet, and brain. It was then that the ghostly figure carrying the big scythe appeared out of the mist.

Luckily for Susan, the Grim Reaper was standing in the parking lot of a convenience store; that traveler's haven of food, fluids, and shelter. She ducked in, downed three hot chocolates, soup, and a couple of donuts. Still shaking, she managed to get back on her bike for the rest of the ride. The black-hooded apparition receded into the shadows, cursing Susan's good fortune and the prolific nature of quick marts.

But finding a store is the easy part. Once there, what should you eat to bring yourself back from the dead? How much carbohydrate and sodium do you need to jump-start your battered body, and what are the most healthful choices with the least fat?

Diagnose the Problem
To know what to buy you have to determine what you need. You're probably dehydrated, so one goal is to chug a quart (4 cups) or more of fluid. Next, replenish your energy stores by stocking up on calories—especially carbohydrate. As a guideline, 600 or more calories with at least

Food for the Cold and Wet

REMEDY	NUTRITION INFO	THE VERDICT
Hot chocolate (small serving/ single envelope)	Calories: 112 Carbos: 25 g Fat: 1 g (8% of calories) Sodium: 102 mg	Drinking lots of hot, sweet liquids can help raise body temperature.
Instant soup (1 serving)	Calories: 60 Carbos: 10 g Fat: 1 g (15%) Sodium: 540 mg	Most convenience stores offer boiling water or cold water and a microwave. Soup will warm you from the inside out. Low in carbs, but a good source of sodium.
Coffee with cream and sugar (1 cup)	Calories: 96 Carbos: 17 g Fat: 3 g (28%) Sodium: 25 mg	If you're a java junkie and it's been 4 or 5 hours since your last fix, your headache may actually be a symptom of caffeine withdrawal. If you're doing an extremely long ride and having trouble staying awake, even old, strong coffee can work wonders.

100 grams of carbohydrate should help rev your motor. Also, a Scottish study found that consuming 1,000 milligrams of sodium with a quart of liquid helps you retain any fluid you drink—so take in some salt.

If you look at the items in "Food for the Cold and Wet," above, and "Food for the Hot and Dry" on pages 48 and 49, you'll probably think we're out of our minds. Hot dogs? Ice cream? Of course you shouldn't eat these fat-laden foods every day. But when you're in extremis, they'll bring you to life faster than Frankenstein's monster. For good health, however, try to hold the percentage of calories from fat to 30 percent or less.

Convenience stores also have ibuprofen to ease the pain, plus life savers like plastic bags for makeshift raingear. And make use of the hand dryer in the bathroom. Still comatose? Spend the last of your change in the phone booth. After all, what are friends for?

Food for the Hot and Dry

REMEDY	NUTRITION INFO	THE VERDICT
Sports drink (Gatorade, 32-oz bottle)	Calories: 200 Carbos: 56 g Fat: 0 g (0% of calories) Sodium: 440 mg	A good source of fluid, carbos, and some sodium. Buy the quart bottle (32 oz), drink as much of it as you can, and use the rest to fill your water bottles.
V-8 juice (11.5-oz can)	Calories: 70 Carbos: 15 g Fat: 0 g (0%) Sodium: 880 mg	If you've been sweating heavily, V-8's high sodium content will help you retain other fluids that you drink. Side benefit: V-8 is packed with vitamins A and C.
Ham and cheese sandwich	Calories: 420 Carbos: 34 g Fat: 22 g (47%) Sodium: 1,700 mg	Sometimes your stomach curdles and your teeth ache at the thought of more sweet snacks. Here's some "real food" with ample carbo, calories, and a big hit of sodium. Only drawback: fat content.
Hot dog with ketchup and relish	Calories: 275 Carbos: 27 g Fat: 14 g (46%) Sodium: 990 mg	Here's another option if you crave "real food." Hot dogs offer a reasonable amount of carbos and sodium. Only drawback: fat content.

13
Five Diets for Five Rides

Different types of rides require different types of nutritional preparation. If you eat for a century as you would for an interval workout, or vice versa, you'll be in trouble. Each type of ride has its own list of nutritional do's and don'ts. The following recommendations come from sports nutritionist Elizabeth Applegate, Ph.D., who explains how, what, and when to eat for some common kinds of cycling.

REMEDY	NUTRITION INFO	THE VERDICT
Bean burrito (5 oz)	Calories: 240 Carbos: 45 g Fat: 5 g (19%) Sodium: 580 mg	Here's a satisfying meal, with a good dose of carbohydrate, some sodium, and limited fat.
Gummy bears (3-oz package), red licorice (3 oz)	Calories: 260 Carbos: 62 g Fat: 0 g (0%) Sodium: 20 mg	Pure carbohydrate, easily and quickly absorbed. Not great for your teeth, but at times like this, even your dentist will forgive you.
Fig-bar cookies, cereal bars, crispy rice squares (2-oz package)	Calories: 210 Carbos: 40 g Fat: 4 g (17%) Sodium: 220 mg	A good source of carbo, with limited fat. Toss a pack into your jersey pocket for later.
Snack cakes (package of two cakes)	Calories: 310 Carbos: 56 g Fat: 9 g (26%) Sodium: 380 mg	Snack cakes provide calories and carbo.
Ice cream (one regular cone)	Calories: 320 Carbos: 44 g Fat: 15 g (44%) Sodium: 160 mg	If you're so far gone that the thought of real food has no appeal, ice cream goes down easily and kick-starts the recovery process.
Potato or corn chips (5-oz bag)	Calories: 750 Carbos: 90 g Fat: 45 g (54%) Sodium: 1,125 mg	Gives you a big hit of carbo and sodium, but high in fat.

Commute

Intensity: Steady speed, light to moderate effort

Distance: 5 to 20 miles

Time: Less than 90 minutes

There are two goals in preparing nutritionally for a commute: to ride comfortably, and to have enough energy left when you arrive to do your job or schoolwork.

Eating a preride meal is important. For morning commutes, have a high-carbohydrate breakfast that includes fruit, cereal, fat-free milk, and

whole-grain toast or muffins. For lunch or an afternoon snack, eat nutritious foods such as pasta, fruits, and vegetables so that your glycogen
stores are fully replenished for the ride home. Avoid eating sugary foods
an hour before cycling if you find that they create hypoglycemia (fa-
tiguing changes in your blood sugar level).

Don't let your commuting get in the way of maintaining a balanced
diet. For example, don't overdo carbo at the expense of sufficient protein. This could lead to long-term performance problems and even affect your health.

In general, give yourself 30 to 45 minutes to digest your meal before
you begin pedaling. Caffeine (coffee, tea, cola) might give you that get-
up-and-go feeling, but it's also a diuretic. Large amounts will cause
your body to expel fluid and magnify the losses you incur while riding,
which will reduce performance. In fact, fluid replacement should be
your primary refueling concern during a commute. One bottle of fluid
per hour should be sufficient. Drink more if it's extremely hot and
humid.

Middle Distance

Intensity: Moderate basic training ride

Distance: 15 to 50 miles

Time: 90 minutes to 3 hours

Nutritionally, there are two dangers to avoid on training rides. The
first is allowing yourself to bonk. Glycogen stores can become depleted
on rides that last more than 2 hours. The second is dehydration, the loss
of body fluid that results in sluggishness and fatigue. You can avoid both
conditions by using a sports drink. It will supply glucose and liquid simultaneously in a form that is quickly usable by your body. Make sure
that you maintain a steady supply by sipping every 10 to 15 minutes.

Avoid fatty foods prior to training rides. Things like pastries, chocolate, or cream cheese take time to digest and contain less readily available fuel. Instead, eat a high-carbohydrate meal or snack. Remember
that carbohydrate should make up 60 to 65 percent of your daily caloric
intake, especially if you ride on consecutive days. Because individual
needs are different, you may want to nibble a high-carbo energy bar
while riding. For a 2-hour outing, 100 to 200 calories should be enough
to prevent any chance of bonking.

About 20 minutes before leaving, drink a tall glass of water. This is important to combat sweat loss during warm weather.

Interval Training

Intensity: Hard efforts interspersed with easy pedaling for recovery

Distance: 10 to 30 miles

Time: 30 minutes to 2 hours

Interval training is the best way to become a stronger, faster cyclist. It's also a great way to burn your muscles with lactic acid. Intense anaerobic riding produces lactic acid within muscles faster than it can be removed, which soon inhibits their ability to contract. Because your circulatory system is responsible for flushing away lactic acid and other metabolites, it's crucial that blood not be confined in your digestive tract when you're doing intervals. To ensure that it won't be, allow 2 to 4 hours for digestion before this type of riding. You should also drink at least 16 ounces of water about an hour beforehand because losses from perspiration will be great.

In addition, drink between every hard effort. You don't need carbo replenishment during interval training unless your total time will exceed 2 hours. If it will, take a sports drink, which is much easier to digest during intense riding than solid food.

Hills

Intensity: Climbing for much of the route

Distance: 10 to 30 miles

Time: $2\frac{1}{2}$ hours or less

A hilly ride is intense enough to burn your carbohydrate reserves. So the key is to plan ahead. Eat a meal of about 600 calories (yogurt, bagel, fruit, low-fat cookies) 2 to 4 hours before your ride.

If you do this and still run low on fuel, experiment with foods and liquids that are high in sugar, such as sports drinks, undiluted fruit juice, and cookies. Ingest them just before you begin the ride and the sugar will usually kick in when your legs begin to fade.

Preride nutrition is especially important for a hilly course because it's difficult to eat on the bike. The best way to replenish energy during the ride is with a sports drink. Take swigs whenever you're descending or when the climbing is moderate enough that you aren't breathing hard.

After the ride, be sure to refuel. This is essential for recovery following any hard effort. If you eat high-carbo foods soon after finishing, your glycogen stores will be back to normal for the next day's ride. Or, you can use one of the commercial drinks known as carbo-loaders. These are easy to digest and replace fluid as well as calories.

Long Distance

Intensity: Low-to-moderate steady pace

Distance: 50 to 100 miles or more

Time: 4 hours or more

You can't survive a long ride on bad nutrition. In fact, when a cyclist struggles in an event such as a century ride, it's usually because of poor eating habits. The solution is good planning before, during, and after the big event.

During a century, you'll probably try to ride at a steady, comfortable pace, which means you'll be burning more fat for energy. Nonetheless, carbohydrate stores are still the limiting factor. Make sure yours are high by eating lots of carbo-rich foods in the days preceding the event. Up your daily calorie intake to at least 70 percent carbohydrate, and increase your fluid intake as well. Stay off the bike or do short and easy rides on the final day or two, and your muscles will be packed with glycogen.

The day of the century, eat a hearty preride meal. A pancake breakfast (light on the butter, of course) with fruit and plenty of water should do the trick. Allow time for at least partial digestion before the start, or full digestion if there will be early hills.

Plan carefully for how and what you'll eat during the ride. Most organized centuries have well-stocked food stops. If not, carry sandwiches made with moderately low-fat ingredients (jam, honey, apple butter, bananas) plus other high-carbo snacks such as cookies or energy bars. Pack your food in small plastic bags that you can open with one hand. Keep these in your jersey's rear pockets and nibble throughout the ride, starting in the first half-hour even if you don't feel hungry. Your body handles a steady intake of small food portions much better than one or two big loads.

Fluid replacement is crucial, of course. Carry at least two bottles so you won't run out between stops. For carbo nourishment, use sports drinks rather than water. Caffeinated beverages, such as some soft drinks, may provide a physical and mental boost late in a long ride, but research shows that caffeine has much less effect if you're a routine daily user.

As soon as possible after a long ride, begin replenishing your exhausted glycogen stores by consuming carbo-rich foods and drinks. This is essential if you plan to ride again the next day. Then, if you want to toast your great achievement with a glass of champagne, go ahead. It's best to wait until your postride reloading is done, because alcohol can interfere with glycogen refueling and you body's fluid balance.

14
Relief for a Queasy Stomach

It can happen anytime—at the crest of a steep hill, during an impromptu training sprint, at the start of an important race, or during a long ride in hot weather. Suddenly, your stomach doesn't feel so good. Although the queasiness usually passes, it sometimes can leave you retching.

Experts agree that exercise-induced nausea is most likely to occur among novice riders or those trying to get back in shape after a long layoff. Says James Stray-Gunderson, M.D., who works in the Human Performance Lab at the University of Texas Southwestern, "It's a common thing, but the fitter you get, the less it tends to happen. However, even fit people, if they're really going for it, can become nauseated and throw up."

Scientists aren't sure of all the causes, but they list the following as the main culprits.

■ A stomach that empties slowly. Both exercise and digestion require increased blood flow. When you ride with a lot of food or fluid in your belly, your stomach and working muscles battle for extra blood. And "your muscles always win," says dietitian Evelyn Tribole, a spokesperson for the American Dietetic Association. The result is that food doesn't leave the stomach as quickly as it should, and nausea may occur.

According to George Brooks, Ph.D., a professor of exercise physiology at the University of California at Berkeley, it's when your intensity approaches 75 to 80 percent of your max VO$_2$—your maximum aerobic ability—that blood is shunted away from your stomach. Since training improves your oxygen uptake, Dr. Brooks explains that being fit "allows you to exercise harder and still move food through." He also suspects that gastric emptying may improve with training. In other words, the more you ride while eating and drinking, the more efficient your digestive system becomes.

■ Irritation of the stomach lining. Brian Maxwell, a former world-class marathoner and a co-originator of the PowerBar, says that exercise-related nausea can be caused by liquid sloshing in the stomach for long periods, which irritates the mucous membrane. While road riders would be far less susceptible than runners (who do have a higher rate of nausea and vomiting), this could be an important factor for mountain bikers.

Maxwell says that eliminating this possible cause was part of the rationale behind adding oat bran to PowerBars. Theoretically, soluble fiber absorbs water, expands to an easily digestible gel, then slowly releases water and nutrients into the bloodstream.

■ A lower pH. According to Dr. Stray-Gunderson, vigorous riding exhausts the energy substrates—or fuel—in cells and produces acids. If your level of exercise is so high that your body is unable to buffer these acids, your pH level will fall, triggering nausea, headache, restlessness, and weakness.

■ Dehydration. Being dry can compound the problem of lowered pH. If you are insufficiently hydrated to produce sweat for vital body cooling, the necessary fluid will be pulled from your blood. Thus, the pH effect worsens. As Dr. Stray-Gunderson explains, "You don't have enough blood to absorb and buffer the acids being produced."

In addition, dehydration alone can cause nausea. The process is a vicious cycle. If you're riding in hot weather and don't drink enough, you'll certainly become dehydrated and possibly nauseated. Once your stomach is upset, you won't want to put anything in it (particularly warm water), so the problem is compounded.

■ Anxiety. Those pre-event jitters can stress your stomach just as much as high-intensity exercise and heat. And according to dietitian Ellen Coleman, an exercise physiologist and marathon athlete, "Whenever you stress the gastrointestinal system, it slows down." Because digestion isn't a priority in an emergency (such as an impending race), the brain slows stomach contractions, which impedes digestion. It isn't surprising, then, that a nervous cyclist with food and fluid in his stomach might get nauseated.

There are other, more obvious causes of nausea, including excessive alcohol consumption the night before a long ride or a race, too much caffeine (especially if you aren't accustomed to it), rich foods, food poisoning, and even flu. If you find that nausea is a chronic problem when you ride, there may be something more serious at work, and you should consult a physician.

Simple Solutions

If you're a hard-charger, occasional nausea may be inevitable. Often, however, it can be avoided by following a few simple precautions.

■ Eat sensibly the night before a hard ride. Ingest nonspicy, high-carbohydrate foods and little or no alcohol and caffeine.

■ Eat lightly before an event. Tribole recommends a small meal of 500 to 700 calories 3 hours before the start. This might consist of a bowl of oatmeal with fat-free milk, a banana, and a raisin English muffin. Or eat a 200-calorie snack, such as four graham crackers or a slice of raisin bread and a glass of juice, 1 to 2 hours prior to the ride.

■ Before and during the ride, avoid foods high in fat or insoluble fiber. These are difficult to digest and stay in the stomach longer. Instead, eat foods that are easily digestible and rich in complex carbohydrate, such as bread, cereal, muffins, crackers, pretzels, and pasta.

Don't eat anything solid within 30 minutes of a big climb. It won't have time to digest, and will sit like a lump in your stomach as blood is pulled into hard-working muscles.

■ Avoid highly acidic foods such as citrus fruits, which can exacerbate the problem of lowered pH. If you become nauseated after using citrus-flavored sports drinks, try a different flavor.

■ If you're doing an especially long ride, practice eating and drinking during your training so that your stomach gets used to digestion during exercise.

■ Use training rides to test foods and fluids so that you can eliminate those that create problems. Never experiment during an important event.

■ For rides of 2 to 4 hours, sports drinks with a carbohydrate concentration of 5 to 8 percent are adequate. For longer rides, higher concentrations may be more beneficial. Again, experiment during training to learn whether your stomach is affected. Select drinks made with glucose polymer or maltodextrin, which are more readily absorbed than simple sugar solutions. Fructose causes stomach upset in some riders.

■ Stay hydrated by drinking lots of water in the days preceding the event. If you're awake early enough on the day of the ride, consume about 20 ounces 3 hours before the start. Then, just 5 minutes prior to riding, drink another 10 to 15 ounces.

■ During the event, don't wait until you're thirsty to drink. Instead, drink at preplanned intervals. Four ounces of fluid every 15 minutes should be enough unless it's hot and humid.

■ Cool water is more palatable and better absorbed. The night before your ride, chill one of your water bottles and freeze the other for a steady source of cool fluids.

■ After the ride, rehydrate with plenty of cool liquids. Stay away from alcoholic beverages for several hours because they act like diuretics.

■ Clean your bottles after each ride, particularly if you use sports drinks. Don't risk sickness by using a bottle that shows signs of mold inside.

15
How to Control Binge Eating

Admit it. There have been times when you've gotten off the bike and consumed anything you could get your hands on. A bag of cookies. A handful of candy bars. A quart of ice cream. Aisle 5 at the supermarket.

Though not uncommon, postride binges can be unsettling because you're probably careful about what you eat otherwise. So what causes these feeding frenzies and, more important, how can you control them? Nancy Clark, author of *Nancy Clark's Sports Nutrition Guidebook*, provides some answers.

Q: *What causes postride binges?*

A: When you start overeating, it's usually because you're physiologically starving. When you get hungry, your body craves quick energy, which generally is sweets. And when you're really hungry and tired and feeling you deserve to eat because you've just ridden for 2 hours, it's easy to overdo it.

Q: *Why do some riders get so hungry?*

A: For a lot of people, a big motivation to exercise is losing weight. If you're riding hard—say 20 mph—you might be burning 11 calories per minute. If you're out for 60 minutes, that's 660 calories—a lot of food. If all you've had beforehand is a 200-calorie breakfast, you won't have much control when you spot an ice cream store afterward. To prevent these binges, simply have a bigger breakfast. That way, you'll have the presence of mind to eat appropriately afterward.

Q: *What constitutes a big breakfast?*

A: In studies, subjects who ate 400 to 1,200 calories of carbohydrate 1 to 4 hours before exercising were able to prolong their endurance. What, when, and how much you eat depends on what works for you. I stress high-carbohydrate, low-fat foods and give these general guidelines for when and how much to eat: 3 to 4 hours before exercising, consume 700 to 800 calories; 2 to 3 hours before, consume 200 to 400 calories; 1 to 2 hours before, consume up to 400 calories in liquid form if possible; less than 1 hour before, consume 100 to 200 calories.

Q: *What if you ride in the late afternoon or evening?*

A: Make sure you have a good breakfast and lunch. A preride snack may also be in order.

Q: *Some veteran riders claim that their metabolism has adapted to cycling, and they can conserve food better on the bike. Is this possible?*

A: Yes, and I think it happens when the body doesn't have fat to lose. As people get down toward their setpoint (optimum body fat percentage), they begin to get a little more energy efficient.

Q: *Won't eating on the bike help stave off that ravenous hunger?*

A: Yes. If you're cycling for more than 90 minutes, it's helpful to eat something during the ride. Some cyclists use sports drinks. Some drink water and eat bananas, energy bars, or whatever else appeals to them. What you're looking for is fluid and carbohydrate. With a sports drink, you get both in one bottle.

Q: *Why do some cyclists crave particular foods after a ride?*

A: Usually, when you need quick energy, you crave sweets. If you're in a real calorie deficit, you may also crave fat. Common cravings like ice cream and cookies are really just a combination of the two. Sometimes, when you eat too much carbohydrate before an event, you crave protein afterward. A craving for salty foods means that's what your body needs. And if you crave or chew ice, that's often a sign of iron deficiency.

Q: *Some cyclists aren't hungry immediately after riding but become ravenous a few hours later. Why?*

A: You get really hot during exercise, and when your body temperature is elevated, it can kill your appetite. When your body temperature gets down to a more normal level, your appetite returns. When swimmers come out of the water, they tend to be ravenous because they're cold.

Q: *What's the best way to eat when the postride hungries hit?*

A: Your hunger is real, so you need to give your body what it wants in terms of recovery food, and that's carbohydrate. For casual riders, it's not that big a factor because they don't deplete their glycogen stores. But the harder you exercise, the more important your recovery diet becomes. I recommend 0.5 gram of carbohydrate per pound of body weight within 2 hours after a workout, and then the same amount again 2 hours later. If you weigh 150 pounds, that's 75 grams of carbohydrate or 300 calories, an amount you can get from a cup of orange juice and a bagel or a bowl of cereal with a banana.

Q: *Can a bit of frivolous eating hurt after a ride?*

A: If you're eating more than 1,800 calories a day and 10 percent of those are sugar, it's still within reason. A 180-calorie treat isn't going to cause you to die of nutritional deficiencies. There's something to be said for reward foods—we're all human. Just make sure that in general you have a good, wholesome diet.

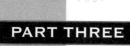

PART THREE

Weight Control

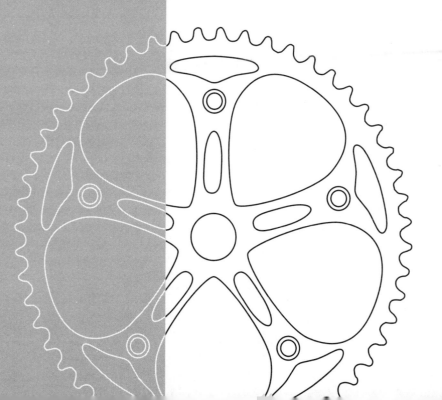

16

The Skinny on Body Fat

Fat. It's a three-letter "four-letter word." Excess body fat can be harmful to health, and packing extra pounds on hills turns you into an anchor on a bike. Consider this: If a fit 165-pound rider loses 10 pounds but retains the same power, that person will save 2 minutes on a 5-mile, 6-percent climb.

That's a great incentive for trimming body fat. On the other hand, you could also become skinny to the point of weakness and poor performance. To investigate this issue, here are answers to the most common questions received from the readers of *Bicycling* magazine.

What body fat percentage is best?

Body fat levels of elite endurance athletes range from 5 to 9 percent in men and 12 to 20 percent in women. These are much lower than general population averages of 15 percent in men and 27 percent in women. Cycling performance will improve with fat loss, but only to a point. How low you can safely go varies among individuals. The leanest cyclist isn't necessarily the fastest.

In pro cycling, extreme leanness is in vogue, particularly for climbers. It's widely believed that Bjarne Riis's relentless dieting was a factor in his 1996 Tour de France victory. Former road pro Bob Roll says, "Ever since Riis, no one in the pro ranks will eat anymore. It used to be you just avoided heavy cream. Now the directors won't even let you use salad dressing."

Unfortunately, it's not that simple. There's a fine line between optimal performance and deteriorating performance.

Can you be too lean?

Yes. Severely limiting food intake to lose body fat can disturb the body's hormonal balance. This should be of particular concern to women, who are susceptible to the downward spiral known as female athlete triad. This includes disordered eating, amenorrhea (missing menstrual periods), and osteoporosis (bone loss). Some athletes in their twenties have the bones of 70- or 80-year-olds, putting them at higher risk for fractures now and in the future.

And men, that Y chromosome lurking in your genes doesn't protect you. Excessive dieting can lower testosterone levels, reducing fertility and libido—and putting your bones at risk, too.

Do we need body fat?

Yes. We couldn't live without it. "Essential fat" needed to sustain life is found in the brain and central nervous system, bone marrow, cell membranes, women's breast tissue, and other organs. Essential fat represents about 3 percent of body weight in men and 8 percent in women. Fat is also an important energy source. A 140-pound adult with 15 percent body fat has about 85,000 calories of stored fat, enough to live on for a month.

How much body fat is too much?

Obesity increases your risk of heart disease, diabetes, high blood pressure, and some types of cancer. But people who are "fit and fat" don't seem to be at high risk. Research done at the Cooper Clinic for Aerobics Research in Houston showed that normal-weight couch potatoes are at greater risk than fit, overweight individuals.

It also matters where the extra fat is carried. So-called apples are at much higher risk than pears. The former describes excess fat in the stomach area and is more common in men. A waist circumference greater than 39 inches is a clear sign. The latter is marked by excess fat in the hips and thighs and is more common in women.

How is body fat measured?

Body fat can't be measured directly, only estimated. Even the best methods have errors of 3 percentage points or more. So if you're told you have 12 percent body fat, you could have anywhere from 9 to 15 percent.

What are the most common measurement methods?

There are five choices: underwater weighing, which measures body density (denser bodies have less fat); skinfold measurement, which assesses the thickness of fat located under the skin; bioelectrical impedance analysis, a measure of how much electric current passes through the body, which indicates body water that, in turn, reflects lean tissue; near-infrared interactance, which measures optical density at the biceps; and dual-energy x-ray absorptiometry, which measures bone mineral density but can also differentiate between fat and lean tissue.

All of these tests, with the exception of the skinfold method, are conducted in a lab. Check with your physician to find out what's available in your area.

What's the bottom line?

Optimizing your body's fat content can help your cycling performance and your health. But don't get obsessed about exact percentages because they probably aren't quite accurate. Talk with a sports medicine physician about your fitness level and goals, and together determine an optimal body fat range for you. Also, use the same measurement method each time in order to gauge your progress consistently.

17
Cycling Calorie Counter

How many calories did you burn on today's ride? It's a simple question that used to be hard to answer with much precision. Granted, you could estimate your caloric consumption according to averages based on weight and speed. But the results were general and didn't account for all the factors that can affect cycling.

This chapter will change that. You'll be able to calculate how many calories you burn on a specific ride. By factoring in terrain, wind, riding position, and drafting as well as speed and body weight, you'll arrive at the best estimation of caloric expenditure ever devised for cyclists. If you're counting calories as a way to maintain or lose weight, this is your formula for success.

A New Method

Calories are stores of energy contained within the three main food compounds—carbohydrate, fat, and protein. Your body breaks down these compounds and uses a portion of the resulting energy to power the basic physiological processes of life. Simply put, you burn calories just being alive. In fact, during normal daily activities, the rate is about 0.01 calorie per pound of body weight per minute. So if you weigh 150 pounds, you burn approximately 1.5 calories per minute, or 2,160 calories in 24 hours.

The remainder of the energy is either stored as body weight or used to contract muscles for additional movement or exercise. The choice is yours. Accumulate about 3,500 unused calories, for instance, and you'll gain 1 pound. But if you ride regularly, your body will consume these extra calories for energy.

During any aerobic exercise, oxygen is required for caloric combustion. Specifically, 1 liter of oxygen is used for every 5 calories burned. Thus, the way physiology labs have traditionally estimated caloric expenditure is by measuring the amount of oxygen consumed.

James Hagberg, Ph.D., and his colleagues at the University of Florida in Gainesville were among the first to take this understanding out of the laboratory and into the real world. Using mobile equipment, they studied the caloric expenditure of cyclists on the road. Now, using their formula and a calculator, you can put this information to work for you.

Baseline Values

SPEED (MPH)	COEFFICIENT (CAL/LB/MIN)	CALORIE EXPENDITURE		
		120 LB	130 LB	140 LB
8	0.0295	3.5	3.8	4.1
10	0.0355	4.3	4.6	5.0
12	0.0426	5.1	5.5	6.0
14	0.0512	6.1	6.7	7.2
15	0.0561	6.7	7.3	7.9
16	0.0615	7.4	8.0	8.6
17	0.0675	8.1	8.8	9.5
18	0.0740	8.9	9.6	10.4
19	0.0811	9.7	10.5	11.4
20	0.0891	10.7	11.6	12.5
21	0.0975	11.7	12.7	13.7
23	0.1173	14.1	15.1	16.4
25	0.1411	16.9	18.3	19.8

NOTE: If your weight is not listed in the table, determine your baseline value by multiplying your weight (in pounds) by the coefficient next to your speed. For instance, if you weigh 165 pounds and rode 17 mph, multiply 165 by 0.0675. The result (11.1) is your baseline value.

Starting Point

First, consult "Baseline Values" to determine your starting point. It's the number that appears where your weight and speed intersect. For instance, if you weigh 150 pounds and averaged 15 mph on the ride you're analyzing, then your baseline value is 8.4. Later, you'll add and subtract from this number depending on the factors that influenced your ride.

If you pedaled at a fairly constant rate throughout the ride, then average speed is suitable for computing baseline value. If there were parts where your speed increased or decreased significantly, however, then divide the ride into several portions and calculate each segment separately.

For instance, on a 3-hour ride, 1 hour might have been spent at 20 mph, another at 18 mph, and a third at 16 mph. Although the average speed is 18 mph, you actually burned more calories than if you had maintained this rate throughout.

		CALORIE EXPENDITURE			
150 LB	**160 LB**	**170 LB**	**180 LB**	**190 LB**	**200 LB**
4.4	4.7	5.0	5.3	5.6	5.9
5.3	5.7	6.0	6.4	6.7	7.1
6.4	6.8	7.2	7.7	8.1	8.5
7.7	8.2	8.7	9.2	9.7	10.2
8.4	9.0	9.5	10.1	10.7	11.2
9.2	9.8	10.5	11.1	11.7	12.3
10.1	10.8	11.5	12.2	12.8	13.5
11.1	11.8	12.6	13.3	14.1	14.8
12.2	13.0	13.8	14.6	15.4	16.2
13.4	14.3	15.1	16.0	16.9	17.8
14.6	15.6	16.6	17.6	18.5	19.5
17.6	18.8	19.9	21.1	22.3	23.5
21.2	22.6	24.0	25.4	26.8	28.2

The reason is simple. As you go faster, air resistance and energy expenditure increase exponentially. Raising your speed 2 mph for 60 minutes gives you a calorie-burning boost that's not entirely offset by decreasing your speed 2 mph for the same period.

Once you have your baseline value, write it on line 1 of the "Calorie Consumption Worksheet." Now, this number must be adjusted based on some key variables.

Surface Area

Air resistance is the biggest obstacle to overcome while riding. An important factor is your surface area—the size of the body you're trying to move through the air. The ideal is to be strong and lean. This way, you have lots of muscle to move minimal surface area.

One study, conducted by *Bicycling* magazine's Fitness Advisory Board member David Swain, Ph.D., quantified the effects of size and surface area. He found that for every pound of body weight greater than 154 pounds, energy expenditure per pound decreased by approximately 0.5

Calorie Consumption Worksheet

Line 1: Baseline Value ± _____

Line 1a: Surface Area Adjustment ± _____

Line 2: ± _____

Line 2a: Terrain Adjustment ± _____

Line 3: = _____

Line 3a: Wind Adjustment ± _____

Line 4: = _____

Line 4a: Riding Position Adjustment + _____

Line 5: = _____

Line 5a: Drafting Adjustment − _____

Grand Totals: Total Calories Burned per Minute ± _____

Total Calories Used for Life Support − _____

Total Minutes of Riding × _____

Total Calories Burned Riding = _____

percent. Conversely, caloric expenditure increased by the same amount for every pound less than 154. This means that, in most cases, heavier riders can generate more power relative to their body weight. They require less energy than lighter riders to overcome air resistance.

To apply this to yourself, calculate the difference between your weight and 154. Halve this difference, then divide by 100. Multiply the resulting number by your baseline value to derive your surface area adjustment. Write it on line 1a of the "Calorie Consumption Worksheet." If you weigh more than 154, subtract this adjustment from your baseline value. If you weigh less, add it. Put the result on line 2.

Terrain

If your ride was mostly flat, put 0 on line 2a and write the same number on line 3 that you did on line 2. Then go to the next section. If your ride was hilly, read on.

Climbing at any speed burns more calories than cycling on flat ground at the same rate. Conversely, when you're descending (even if you pedal), you burn fewer calories than when you're riding on the flats at the same rate. So the question is, do downhills offset uphills?

For most hilly rides, the calories used while climbing and the calories saved when descending almost offset each other, but not quite. So if you rode a hilly out-and-back course, an adjustment is necessary. The reason is that as you climb, you're battling gravity. But as you descend, you don't enjoy the full advantage of this force. Once again, air resistance is to blame because it rises exponentially with speed, making the descent not as quick and easy as the climb is slow and hard.

To derive an accurate measure of caloric expenditure, you need to estimate what percentage of the ride was spent climbing. Then, multiply your adjusted baseline value (line 2) by 0.01 for each 10 percent. For example, if you were climbing for 30 percent of the time, multiply by 0.03. The result is your terrain adjustment. Write it on line 2a and add it to line 2. The sum goes on line 3.

Of course, not every ascent culminates in a descent. A point-to-point ride may have an overall elevation gain. If this describes the ride you're analyzing, multiply your weight by the total number of feet you climbed. The resulting number is in foot/pounds, a measure of work. For instance, if you weigh 150 pounds and took an hour to complete a course with a net elevation gain of 100 feet, you've done 15,000 (150 × 100)

foot/pounds of work. (For precision in measuring vertical gain, the
Cateye AT100 cyclecomputer has an altimeter.)

One foot/pound of work requires 0.0014 calories, so multiply the result by this number, then divide by the total minutes ridden. Using the
same example as before, the result is 0.35 calorie per minute
(15,000 × 0.0014 = 21; 21 ÷ 60 minutes = 0.35). This is the number of
extra calories required per minute to climb the additional 100 feet. Put
the result of your calculations on line 2a, add it to line 2, and write the
sum on line 3.

If you rode a point-to-point course that has an overall decrease in elevation, follow the same steps but subtract the result from line 2.

Wind

If you rode in calm conditions, skip this section, write 0 on line 3a, and
bring down the previous adjusted baseline value to line 4. If it was
windy, however, you'll need to make an adjustment.

Wind, like hills, can make a ride harder or easier. With out-and-back
or loop courses, the energy saved with a tailwind almost offsets the extra
calories burned against a headwind. Wind direction varies, however.
Sometimes the headwind you battle on the ride out isn't equal to the
tailwind you enjoy on the way back, or vice versa. If the wind changed
in this manner during your ride, multiply the adjusted baseline value
(line 3) by 0.03 if the wind was light, 0.04 if it was moderate, or 0.05 if it
was strong. Write the result on line 3a. If the wind was against you most
of the way, add it to the adjusted baseline value on line 3. If it was with
you, subtract it.

If you rode a point-to-point course with either a constant headwind
or tailwind, you need to make a different adjustment. First, halve the
wind speed. If it was a headwind, add this number to your actual speed.
If it was a tailwind, subtract it. The result is your wind-adjusted speed.
Next, refer again to "Baseline Values" on pages 64 and 65 and find the
number that corresponds to the intersection of your weight and wind-
adjusted speed. Subtract your original baseline value (line 1) from this
number. The result is your wind adjustment, which should be entered
on line 3a. Again, if you had a headwind, it should be added to line 3. If
you had a tailwind, it should be subtracted. Tally the result on line 4.

For example, if you weigh 150 pounds and rode 15 mph into a 10-
mph headwind, your wind-adjusted speed is 20 mph (10 divided by 2 +

15) and your wind adjustment is 5 (13.4, the adjusted baseline value −
8.4, the original baseline value). Since it was a headwind, the result is
added to line 3. Conversely, if you weigh 150 pounds and rode 15 mph
with a 10-mph tailwind, your wind adjustment is 3.1 (8.4 − 5.3), which
is subtracted from line 3.

Wind conditions are rarely this distinct, however. A crosswind is
more common than a direct headwind or tailwind. The energy requirement of riding with most crosswinds is about 70 percent that of cycling
into a headwind. To figure your wind adjustment in a crosswind, use the
method described earlier, just as if you had ridden into a headwind.
Then multiply the wind adjustment by 0.7 and add the result to the adjusted baseline value.

For example, if you weigh 150 pounds and rode 15 mph in a 10-mph
crosswind, your wind adjustment is 3.5 (5 × 0.7). Add this to line 3.

Riding Position

At speeds below 15 mph, there's little difference between the caloric cost
of riding in an upright position or low on the drops or on an aero bar.
When you're moving faster, however, a low position burns significantly
fewer calories. Similarly, you expend less energy when your bike is free
of racks, panniers, fenders, and so on, all of which make you less aero-
dynamic.

If you were in a low position for most of the ride, you don't need to
adjust your baseline value. Simply enter the same number on line 5 that
you did on line 4. But if you sat upright most of the time, or if your bike

Adjustment for Riding Position

SPEED (MPH)	INCREASES IN CALORIE EXPENDITURE
15	3
16	8
17	12
18	18
19	22
20	26
22.5	38
25	50

was outfitted with panniers, consult "Adjustment for Riding Position" on page 69. Find your speed and the increase in caloric expenditure listed beside it. Multiply your adjusted baseline value (line 4) by this number, then enter the result on line 4a. Add it to line 4 and write the sum on line 5.

Drafting

Dr. Hagberg's research found that drafting reduces workload by about 1 percent for each mph.

If you didn't draft, or if you rode alone, no adjustment is necessary on your worksheet. But if you drafted another cyclist for the entire ride, you need to turn your speed into a percentage and subtract it from the adjusted baseline value (line 5). For instance, if you rode at 15 mph, take 15 percent of your adjusted baseline value. Write the result on line 5a and subtract it from line 5.

It's more likely, however, that you drafted for only part of the ride. If so, convert your speed from mph to a percentage as before. Then, estimate what fraction of the ride you drafted and, in turn, take that percentage of your adjusted baseline value. For example, if you drafted for a third of a 15-mph ride, take 5 percent (one-third of 15) of line 5. Enter the result on line 5a, then subtract it from line 5. This gives you the total number of calories burned per minute of riding.

Final Adjustment

Because this result includes your body's basic physiological requirements for living, to determine how many calories were used just for riding, you need to make one final adjustment.

Multiply your weight in pounds by 0.01, which is the number of calories per pound that you burn naturally. Subtract the result from total calories burned per minute. Multiply that by the total minutes of riding. The result is the total calories burned while riding. Then, think of all the calories you used just figuring this out.

18
Your Perfect Weight

If I could just lose 10 pounds, I'd climb a lot better." If you haven't chanted this popular mantra yourself, you've probably heard it from friends. And it's true—providing you lose fat rather than muscle. For some cyclists, slimming down can pay off dramatically in performance gains, not to mention better health. Should you consider shedding a few pounds? More important, what's the best way to lose weight—and keep it off?

First, take an objective look at your weight and body composition. Health experts recommend that your body mass index (BMI) be between 19 and 25. BMI is a measure of relative weight calculated by dividing body weight in kilograms by the square of your height in meters. If you aren't mathematically inclined, see "Body Mass Index Calculation" on page 72, which uses inches and pounds.

Health risks from being overweight are believed to increase with a BMI above 27, but there's an important caveat: Research conducted at the Cooper Clinic for Aerobics Research in Houston shows that overweight people who are fit actually have lower death rates than normal or underweight people who are unfit.

Also realize that BMI measurements have a major drawback: They don't reveal body composition. At a given BMI, body fat can vary considerably. For example, someone with a BMI of 26 and a relatively high fat level could improve cycling performance by shedding his excess fat. But a lean, muscular rider with the same BMI probably won't get the same benefit from losing weight. With little fat to lose, any weight that he loses would more likely come from the muscle that propels him down the road.

Unfortunately, commercially available methods of estimating body fat (see chapter 16) aren't especially accurate. This makes an unflinching visual inspection nearly as useful. You don't need to jump up and down in front of a mirror to see if anything jiggles that shouldn't. Instead, stand upright and pinch some skin next to your navel between your thumb (on top) and forefinger (below). If the fold is more than an inch thick, you may be carrying excess fat.

Body Mass Index Calculation

HEIGHT	WEIGHT AT BMI 19 (LB)	WEIGHT AT BMI 25 (LB)	WEIGHT AT BMI 27 (LB)
5'0"	97	128	138
5'1"	100	132	143
5'2"	104	136	147
5'3"	107	141	152
5'4"	110	145	157
5'5"	114	150	162
5'6"	117	155	167
5'7"	121	159	172
5'8"	125	164	177
5'9"	128	169	182
5'10"	132	174	188
5'11"	136	179	193
6'0"	140	184	199
6'1"	144	189	204
6'2"	148	194	210

If your BMI is much above 25, or you know you have fat to lose, consider the advice that follows. Conversely, if your BMI is closer to 19 or 20 and you're interested in going uphill faster, you're better off doing strength training, sticking to a sound training and nutrition program, or even purchasing lightweight components for your bike.

Keys to Weight Loss

Dieting, by itself, doesn't work. In the short term, any diet that decreases caloric intake will result in weight loss. So although new diets appear frequently, in most cases they're simply repackaged strategies that have been tried before. The disheartening truth is that from 2 to 5 years post-diet, most dieters will have regained the lost weight. In fact, they often gain more. Although the exact cause is unknown, it's thought that most diets simply can't be sustained as a permanent lifestyle change. So old eating habits return along with the weight. There are some other points to consider as well.

Exercise is critical. Studies show that people who lose weight by burning excess calories with exercise are much more likely to maintain

How Pros Shave Pounds

Followers of pro road racing have been struck by the extreme leanness of top riders. It's no wonder—studies show that losing weight can result in a performance boost on a par with most banned substances.

Danish pro Bjarne Riis, who ended Spaniard Miguel Indurain's 5-year monopoly on the Tour de France in 1996, looked emaciated, his arms mere pipe stems. Indurain himself came into cycling at 196 pounds but slimmed down to 172 during his prime. Italian Andrea Tafi was third in a recent Paris-Roubaix classic at a reported 176 pounds and 8 percent body fat, but 5 months later, when he won 4 major races in the span of 4 weeks, he was down to 154 and 3.5 percent. And Aussie Patrick Jonker turned into a contender when he went from 163 pounds to 150.

How do already lean pro riders cut weight? Their techniques are closely guarded, but here are a few methods that are rumored to be making the rounds.

- They eat a big breakfast, ride 5 to 7 hours while consuming carbo drinks, eat a high-carbo meal in midafternoon, then eat nothing until the next morning. Theory: The body stores fat more readily at night, so going to bed hungry forces your body to use fat stores while you sleep rather than accumulating more fat.

- They ride hard for 3 to 4 hours before breakfast. Theory: Riding while carbo-deficient forces the body to use fat as fuel.

- They use diet drugs to suppress appetite. Theory: If hunger can be kept at bay, strongly disciplined cyclists can more easily accept the misery of doing long training rides in a glycogen-depleted state.

- They undereat while riding a multiday race, using it for training rather than a good placing. Theory: The stress of competition makes it easier to work hard, and the rider can be closely supervised by team doctors to make sure he adheres to a diet with too few calories.

Are any of these strategies recommended? No. All of these weight-loss methods are extreme and expose a rider to serious dangers including dehydration, lowered performance, snowballing fatigue, and possible cardiac problems. If you need to lose weight, follow the sensible approach of exercise, balanced nutrition, and moderate calorie reduction that is discussed throughout this book.

weight loss. Both aerobic exercise and strength training play a role. Increasing either the intensity or the duration of your cycling workouts increases energy expenditure. Adding resistance training two or three times a week not only increases calorie burning, but the added strength will help you get up that hill faster. Another exercise benefit: It may help prevent dieting-related loss of muscle mass and accompanying decreases in your metabolic rate.

What you eat does matter. Although diets alone don't work, what you eat obviously does matter. Limiting (but not eliminating) fat is important because it appears that we don't regulate fat calories as closely as we do calories from carbohydrate or protein. When carbo or protein intakes are increased, your body responds by increasing their oxidation (use for energy). But increases in fat don't lead to parallel increases in oxidation. It just gets stored on your body.

The lesson is that carbo is key. As a first step, try increasing your fruit and vegetable intake to 10 servings daily. (A serving equals ½ cup of chopped vegetables or a medium-size piece of fruit). This provides great nutrition, lots of fiber, and relatively few calories.

Every meal is important. If you're not a breakfast eater, try to be for 2 weeks. Eating breakfast may prevent overeating later in the day. But don't skimp on dinner, either. One study found that people who ate an inadequate evening meal lost muscle volume, which is an undesirable outcome for cycling.

Monitoring what you eat can lead to success. If you're keeping tabs on your weight, the more frequently you write down what you eat, the more likely you are to lose weight or maintain your weight loss. A diary helps you think twice about whether you're truly hungry or whether you're eating for some unwarranted reason.

Getting support from others helps your cause. Support from family and friends is a crucial element of any lifestyle change. Letting people know your plans increases your accountability and may prevent them from unwittingly sabotaging your efforts.

Shedding pounds takes time. Weight loss should occur at a rate of ½ to 2 pounds per week so that the lost weight isn't valuable muscle tissue. If you lose as much as 10 pounds, maintain the new weight for 6 months before attempting to lose more. This may help your body recognize the new weight as its normal weight and prevent subsequent gain.

19

Winning Tips for Losing Pounds

Cycling is great exercise, but it doesn't make you immune to gaining weight. Just ask Jan Ullrich, the young German star who won the 1997 Tour de France. He gained 20 pounds in the winter after his victory, then struggled the next season to get back to racing weight. It took him the entire spring despite many miles of hard training and competition.

Of course, weight control is a lot easier if you don't get chunky in the first place. If Ullrich had spent more time on winter training and less on the banquet circuit, his metabolism and caloric expenditure would have been higher, keeping away the flab. One common desperation strategy—an ultra-low-calorie crash diet—is simply out of the question because it leaves a person too weak to ride well, and this is certain to undermine motivation.

Maybe you're not in the running for this year's Tour, but if you'd like to get rid of excess weight in a way that also makes you fitter for cycling, use this two-pronged approach: Eat smarter and rev up your exercise program. Here's the right way and the wrong way to do it.

Eat just enough. Don't starve yourself. If you want to keep riding well, you need the strength and stamina that only come from enough carbohydrate and protein. And if you're hungry all the time, you're much more likely to give in to cravings for sweet, high-calorie foods.

Eat foods that make you feel full with fewer calories. Legumes, whole grains, fruits, and vegetables, along with extralean meat, poultry, and fish, are among the most nutritious foods you can eat. They're also more likely to satisfy your hunger even when you eat less.

Burn more than you eat. Stay away from hardcore diets. You may have friends who lost weight on some high-protein, low-fat, or no-carbo diet, but this doesn't mean it will work for you (or even for your friends after a couple of months). There are two keys to weight loss: Burn more calories than you consume, and do it in a way that you can maintain for a lengthy period. If you eat like most people (and you aren't doing high-intensity training), it won't hurt you to cut down on fat and total calories. But you shouldn't eat so little that you feel weak or miserable.

Vary your exercise. Ride hills and add periodic sprints or time trials to your cycling workouts to tax your muscles, boost your heart rate, and increase your calorie consumption.

Weight training helps to increase your metabolism so that you burn more calories even when you're not exercising. It also helps offset the tendency to lose muscle mass along with fat. On the bike, don't subscribe to the popular notion that low-intensity riding burns more fat. The fact is that going harder burns more total calories and is better for weight loss.

Add some meals. Don't skip meals in an attempt to cut calories. You need to keep your blood sugar steady throughout the day to sustain your energy level and prevent cravings for high-fat or sweet snacks.

Eat numerous small meals throughout the day. These can be the three main meals with snacks between, or five or six meals of the same size. This manner of eating provides a constant supply of energy and reduces your urge to eat big meals that overload your system.

Ride a little more. A study of people who successfully lost weight and kept it off for several years found that nearly all of them increased their activity levels while they reduced calories.

Ride your bike an extra half-hour every day. Although the number of calories burned is dependent on your metabolism and workout intensity, you can easily consume an extra 250 a day this way, resulting in the loss of 2 pounds per month—a healthful rate that is easy to sustain.

Be realistic. Trying to lose 20 pounds in a month isn't just difficult, it's unhealthy. And trying to reach such a goal by suddenly quadrupling your mileage is a quick route to overtraining and injury.

Set fitness goals that have nothing to do with weight loss. When members of a New York health club trained to run a marathon, those who did it to improve performance lost weight, while those who did it only because they wanted to lose weight tended to drop out and keep the weight on. Set a goal that will take several months of preparation— riding a century, for example, or an all-day mountain bike ride. Your motivation will be even higher if you get friends to commit to the goal with you.

20
Strategies for the Holidays

For many of us, holidays (and perhaps vacations) mean gluttony followed by a bad case of scale-avoidance and stressful guilt. Indeed, holiday dinners, cookouts, and parties are front-row tickets to these conditions. The predictable pig-outs from Thanksgiving to New Year's Day make for a brisk business in January at fitness clubs and weight-loss clinics.

But keep this in mind: Any upward blip in body weight comes down to a balance of energy. If you eat more calories than you expend, the excess will automatically go into storage in your love handles and other flab-vulnerable places. You just can't fool the First Law of Thermodynamics. What's worse, the off-season holidays dish up an apparently unavoidable and unfortunate double whammy—you're tempted to eat a lot but you can't ride it off.

Here's the good news: There are ways to enjoy good food with family and friends without looking like Santa at the end of it all—and without putting a damper on everyone else's eating exploits. The key is to plan ahead rather than try to undo the damage after the fact. Think tactics. Plan strategies. Know fast moves for unexpected situations. Here are some proven methods to help you come up with a successful game plan.

Eat beforehand. Never arrive hungry at a major eating occasion. If you're starving by the time the food is on the table, you'll want to eat anything that doesn't bite you first. Instead, snack before you get to the big feed. If possible, do some exercise during the day to help balance the calories you'll be ingesting.

Mend the menu. Just as you carry healthful foods and fluids on a long ride, make sure that wholesome alternatives are at hand during the holiday feast. If you are the host or hostess, put the emphasis on choice. Balance fat-laden seasonal traditions with equally delicious and less calorific treats. If you're a guest, offer to bring veggies and low-fat dip or a fruit salad. With some smart choices, you can save 1,000 calories or more at a single party. Over the course of the winter holidays, this can add up to several pounds of ballast you won't be lugging up the hills when spring comes.

Keep your distance. Positioning plays a crucial role in who wins the sprint at the end of a race, and it's just as important for winning the weight-loss war. Don't get boxed in near the buffet table, where the array of food is within easy reach. Instead, sprint in, grab your chow, and jockey to the back of the pack.

Know thyself. Good cyclists know their strengths and weaknesses. This also applies to holiday treats. Can you eat just one? Some of us can, others can't. If you can apply the brakes, by all means have one of whatever you fancy—and savor it. But if you know that once you start there's no stopping, you're probably better off not beginning at all, especially in situations when unlimited quantities are available.

Schedule the next meal. It's important to refuel your muscles after a hard ride—and it's just as important to plan what you eat following a major pork-out. One typical strategy is to avoid eating again for as long as possible. Don't do it. This mistake sets you up for yet another feeding frenzy when hunger takes control. Instead, start the next morning with a light breakfast (cereal, yogurt, fresh fruit) and eat sensibly the rest of the day.

Find substitutes for food. Instead of focusing holiday social gatherings on eating, try something else. If you're on the office party planning committee, plan to go skating or hiking or play volleyball instead of eating cake by the photocopier. If you're getting together with cycling friends, consider riding from dinner to dessert. You'll probably find that it's a welcome relief from food.

Remember that you won't be able to win every round of a holiday food-a-thon. It all goes back to strategy. If you know you're going to overindulge at Thanksgiving dinner or that picnic on the Fourth of July, plan around it by being conservative in the adjoining meals. Don't obsess and diminish the fun of festive times and good food. Holidays are stressful enough as it is.

21

The Case for Fast Riding

Every winter, the same things conspire to make you just a little chubbier: bad weather, minimal daylight, holiday feasts, and the gravitational pull of the couch. Suddenly, you find you've gained several unwanted pounds. Welcome to the ranks of the average North American.

How can you avoid moving up to the next larger size of cycling shorts? First, acknowledge that weight loss doesn't occur overnight. Despite the claims of tabloid diets, the only way to lose 10 pounds in 24 hours is to give birth. To get a svelte climber's physique, you need a structured program of increased activity and a sensible diet. But questions remain whether high- or low-intensity exercise is best, and whether the diet should be high or low in carbohydrate. Here, the myths are laid to rest.

Faster Is Better

Many cyclists remain confused about the optimal exercise intensity for weight loss. Current folk wisdom has it that low-intensity activity burns fat better because fat is the body's primary fuel for slower-paced exercise. While the last part of this statement is true, a study conducted at Georgia State University in Atlanta shows that weight loss depends on the total number of calories burned during a workout, not whether those calories came from carbohydrate or fat.

To illustrate, consider George and Jennifer. They're both trying to shed their spare tires by following moderately high-carbohydrate diets. For our purposes, assume that their body weights, calorie intakes, and fitness levels are equal. George is an advocate of low-intensity exercise and cycles easily for 2 hours, burning 600 calories—with more than half of those calories coming from fat. Meanwhile, Jennifer cycles at high intensity for only 1 hour but also burns 600 calories, mostly from carbohydrate stored in her body as glycogen.

During the rest of the day, George uses carbohydrate as fuel for routine activities as a consequence of his slower workout. But because Jennifer used more of her limited carbo supply for exercise, her body taps into abundant fat stores.

After a few weeks of this routine, both will have lost the same amount of body fat. Note, however, that if Jennifer exercises as long as George, but does so at her high-intensity pace, she'll come out ahead in terms of fat loss.

The bottom line is that the total number of calories expended per day is what counts. If you want to lose weight but have time limitations—and who doesn't in the short days of winter?—ride harder.

Leaner Is Better

The importance of carbohydrate for athletes was virtually undisputed until the appearance of The Zone diet, which advocates a diet that is only 40 percent carbohydrate but a high 30 percent protein and 30 percent fat. The book's recommended diet claims to provide benefits such as weight loss and improved physical performance. Most scien-

Lower Fat, Higher Satisfaction

Here's a comparison of higher- and lower-fat diets. By reducing fat, you get to eat more: more cereal, a snack, a second helping, or dessert. The lower-fat menu also has more protein, vitamins, and fiber.

Higher-Fat Menu (1,500 calories, 40% from fat)

Breakfast: 1 cup coffee, ¼ cup granola, ½ cup whole milk

Lunch: Tuna sandwich on whole-wheat kaiser bun (2 teaspoons margarine, 2 ounces tuna, ¼ cup chopped celery, 1 tablespoon mayonnaise), apple, café latte (made with whole milk)

Dinner: Stir-fry (2 ounces lean beef, ½ cup carrots, ½ cup broccoli, 1 teaspoon soy sauce), ½ cup brown rice, 1 cup green salad, 1 tablespoon blue cheese salad dressing

Lower-Fat Menu (1,500 calories, 15% from fat)

Breakfast: 1 cup coffee, 1 cup toasted oat cereal, ½ cup 1% milk, 1 banana

Lunch: Tuna sandwich (same as above but with 1 teaspoon margarine instead of 2 teaspoons, and 1 tablespoon fat-free dressing instead of mayonnaise), apple, café latte (made with fat-free milk)

Snack: 6 ounces fat-free fruit yogurt

Dinner: Stir-fry (same as above but with 1 teaspoon oil for frying), 1 cup brown rice, 1 cup green salad, 1 teaspoon balsamic vinegar or fat-free dressing

Dessert: Small piece of angel food cake, ½ cup fresh strawberries

tists are skeptical, however—the research simply doesn't support such outcomes.

Studies do show that weight loss occurs at similar rates when subjects are fed high- or low-carbohydrate diets—as long as their diets contain an equal number of calories. But research at Cornell University in Ithaca, New York, makes the case that a higher-fat diet may lead to increased calorie consumption overall. For 11 weeks, volunteers ate as much as they wanted of diets that were either higher in fat (37 percent of calories) or lower in fat (22 percent). Menus for the two diets were identical and included similar-tasting higher- and lower-fat versions of the same foods. On the lower-fat diet, subjects ate fewer calories and lost an average of 5.5 pounds—double the loss of the subjects on the higher-fat diet.

So, just as total calorie expenditure is the bottom line for exercise intensity, total calories eaten is the bottom line for your diet. By limiting (not eliminating) dietary fat, you can cut calories without cutting nutrition. You'll also maintain the carbohydrate needed to fuel high-intensity exercise and keep the volume of food high enough to prevent hunger pangs. So enjoy the pasta but go easy on the olive oil.

22
An Ideal Daily Diet

The world is piled high with calories at every turn—a glutton's dream come true. "Fast" and "convenient" are the mantras, whether it's burger joints, gourmet food, or ethnic eateries tempting you on the streets. Then there are the cookies and chips in your cupboard and the packaged entrees stockpiled in your freezer. Finding the ideal diet, much less the time to prepare it, can seem like an impossible quest. To help you through the maze, here's a list of intelligent, quick-and-easy meals, with the reasoning behind each one.

This ideal dietary day is designed for a 40-year-old male cyclist who weighs 180 pounds and rides for an hour each day. He needs approximately 3,400 calories daily, plus another 800 for his hour of cycling. A 130-pound woman should decrease daily portions by 25 percent and eliminate the evening snack. If you're maintaining your weight and feeling energetic, you can be sure you're getting the right number of calories.

Breakfast (775 calories)

- Toasted multigrain bagel with apricot jam
- 1½ cups bran flakes
- One medium sliced banana
- 1 cup fat-free milk

News headlines vary widely on how diet affects conditions such as heart disease, cancer, high blood pressure, and osteoporosis—but four nutritional constituents (fiber, low fat, fruits, vegetables) have withstood the test of time. In general, your daily diet should include at least 25 grams of fiber, obtained through whole grains, beans, and lots of fruits and veggies. These high-fiber foods are also low in fat, so eat up. They help reduce room for fat intake, which should be no more than 25 to 30 percent of calories. Plus, fruits and vegetables provide vitamins and minerals.

Morning Snack (400 calories)

- cup low-fat fruit yogurt
- One large oatmeal cookie

To function well throughout the day, you need to eat and drink frequently. A general guideline is not to go more than 4 hours during the day without a bite. If you're up with the birds and eat a late lunch, you'll need a midmorning snack. If you train after work and don't eat dinner until you've ridden, showered, shopped for food, driven home, and pushed the buttons on the microwave, you should also snack in midafternoon. (Ideally, allow a couple of hours between eating and a workout to let your stomach empty and the nutrients be absorbed.) One other benefit of snacking: You won't be famished at regular meals. You'll want less then, which usually means you'll eat fewer total calories every day.

Lunch (700 calories)

- Black bean soup mix (add hot water)
- Chicken wrap (large tortilla, cream cheese, salsa or hoisin sauce, large lettuce leaf, 2 ounces of sliced chicken, chopped raw cucumbers, tomatoes)

- Five raw baby carrots

- Orange

- Rice Krispies square

Meals should include at least 3 food groups and a variety of un-processed foods to meet your energy and dietary needs. This meal has foods from the bread and cereal group (tortilla), fruit group (orange), veggie group (baby carrots, cucumber, tomato), and protein group (black beans, chicken). Remember that taking a multivitamin/mineral supplement can help a good diet meet full nutritional requirements, but it can't make up for a substandard diet.

Afternoon Snack (325 calories)

- Two rye crackers

- 1½ ounces Swiss cheese

- 1 cup apple juice

Even moderate dehydration can lessen cycling performance, increase fatigue, and leave you with a headache. Keep a water bottle with you at work, and sip frequently. The apple juice in this snack counts toward fluid intake, as do milk and noncaffeinated beverages.

Dinner (1,000 calories)

- Beef-tofu stir fry (3 ounces lean beef, 2 ounces firm tofu, ½ cup broc-coli, ½ cup mixed red and green peppers, 1½ teaspoons sesame oil, 1 teaspoon soy sauce, 1½ cups brown rice)

- Salad (1 cup romaine lettuce, 2 teaspoons salad dressing)

- Apple crisp with walnuts and raisins (½ cup)

Dinner includes lots of veggies, some protein (from beef and tofu), and carbohydrate from the rice to fuel tomorrow's ride.

Evening Snack (275 calories)

- Toasted English muffin with peanut butter

And that's it: a day's menu with about 3,500 calories (61 percent from carbohydrate, 22 percent from fat) and more than 100 percent of the Recommended Dietary Allowance (RDA) for all vitamins and minerals. It also meets guidelines for fiber, fruit, and vegetable intake.

23
Guidelines for Vegetarians

If you look at a restaurant menu, pick up a food magazine, or tour a grocery store, you can't help noticing the increasing array of vegetarian options. Although only about 4 percent of North Americans consider themselves vegetarians, many more go meatless one or more days per week. Is vegetarian eating healthful? Will it help you become a better rider? There aren't any simple answers.

The health consequences of avoiding meat depend on the quality of your entire diet. Some vegetarian cyclists try to subsist on bagels, pasta, and bananas. That's a mistake. Instead, it's necessary to eat a variety of foods and follow the guidelines in this chapter. When a vegetarian diet is properly designed, it can mean positive health benefits such as lower rates of obesity and heart disease.

Then comes the big question: How will a vegetarian diet affect your cycling? Surprisingly little research has been done on this issue. In one study, Danish researchers compared a meat-containing diet to a vegetarian diet in eight male endurance athletes—four of whom were cyclists. Both diets contained 58 percent carbohydrate, 14 percent protein, and 28 percent fat—proportions recognized as nearly ideal for athletes. Two of the subjects had better endurance after the veggie diet, and six performed worse—but the difference was not statistically significant.

Relatively few high-level racers are vegetarians. This shouldn't come as a surprise, considering that meatless diets are still uncommon among the general population. But peak performances can certainly be achieved on a veggie diet. For example, consider Laurie Brandt Hauptmann, a three-time winner of the Leadville Trail 100 (a grueling mountain bike race at elevations over 10,000 feet). She occasionally uses eggs and dairy products but relies on sponsor Shaklee's powdered soy products for some of the 90 grams of daily protein she needs. She also supplements her diet with vitamins and minerals including calcium, zinc, and antioxidants.

Of course, as it does with Hauptmann, "vegetarian" means different things to different people. Some vegetarians abstain from red meat but eat poultry and fish, while pure vegans avoid all animal products—in-

Meatless Menu

Here's a 1-day vegetarian diet that provides about 2,600 calories and meets all recommended nutritional needs for adult men and women. It has 61 percent of calories from carbohydrate, 26 percent from fat, and 13 percent from protein. It also meets protein recommendations for endurance athletes weighing up to 155 pounds. (Larger cyclists would presumably consume more food, which would provide more protein.) Vegans could substitute soy products for dairy ingredients.

Breakfast: 1 cup whole-grain, ready-to-eat cereal; ¼ cup raisins; 1 cup fat-free milk; 1 cup orange juice

Lunch: Sandwich made with two slices of whole-wheat bread, 2 tablespoons of peanut butter, and one medium banana; five carrot sticks; one large oatmeal cookie; 1 cup fruit or vegetable juice

Snack: One Rice Krispies square

Dinner: One bowl of three-bean chili topped with 1 ounce of Cheddar cheese; 1 cup rice; 1 cup broccoli

Dessert or snack: 1 cup frozen yogurt; ¼ cup cashews; 2 tablespoons chocolate syrup

cluding foods containing honey or gelatin. The nutritional benefits (and challenges) of these different eating patterns vary.

Semi-vegetarian

Semi-vegetarians exclude red meat but may include fish, poultry, and dairy. There are few nutritional concerns with such a diet, although iron deficiency is possible because red meat is the richest source of heme iron—a form that is particularly well-absorbed.

Lacto-ovo vegetarian

Lacto-ovo vegetarians exclude all flesh foods but include dairy products and eggs. The advantage: Dairy products are important sources of protein, calcium, vitamin D, and vitamin B_{12}. (But choose fat-free or low-fat varieties so that your fat intake remains reasonable.) To meet iron needs (especially important for women), dried peas and beans as well as fortified cereals should be included. Any foods prepared in cast-iron cookware also provide traces of iron. Zinc may also be in short supply, because meat and shellfish are the best sources. Substitutes include kidney and pinto beans, dairy products, whole grains, and nuts.

Vegan

Vegans exclude all foods derived from animals. Vegan diets are very low in saturated fat, have no cholesterol, and are usually high in fiber. Challenges include obtaining calcium, vitamin D, and vitamin B_{12}. One way is to use products fortified with these nutrients, such as soy beverages and some breakfast cereals. Many energy bars are also fortified (check labels), though some contain milk protein and may be unacceptable to vegans. There's no effective plant source of vitamin B_{12}. Seaweed has the vitamin, but the most recent research indicates that it is in a form the body can't use. Deficiency symptoms include anemia and neurological problems. Body stores of B_{12} that are developed before a person adopts a vegan diet will last several years, but if the deficiency progresses to include neurological symptoms it can be irreversible. Vegans must also be concerned about zinc and iron, so follow the same recommendations as for lacto-ovo vegetarians.

Protein Is Plentiful

Although vegetarians often worry about protein, it's unwarranted. If you consume enough calories to meet energy needs, you'll generally meet protein requirements, too. Just be sure to replace traditional protein sources with alternatives, don't merely delete them. Also, it's not necessary to combine different protein sources at the same meal to ensure a high-quality intake. Simply eat a variety of protein sources during the day, such as cereal and milk at breakfast and three-bean chili for dinner. Grains, legumes, and dairy products are excellent sources of protein.

In a nutshell, many scientists contend that the positive health benefits of a vegetarian diet arise primarily from what vegetarians eat more of (grains, legumes, nuts, seeds, vegetables, fruits) rather than what they eat less of (primarily meat). Anyone can benefit from including more plant foods in their diet, whether or not they choose to avoid meat.

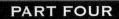

PART FOUR

Special Nutrition

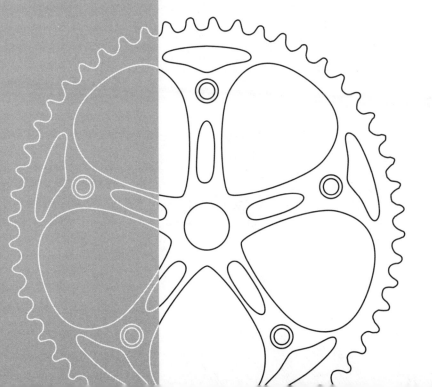

24
The Wonders of Water

Water: the forgotten nutrient. You could survive for years on your current vitamin B_{12} stores, more than a month without food, and a lifetime without nonalcoholic beer—but only days without water. And if your definition of survival is "optimal cycling performance," then the time frame shrinks to hours or less.

You know the saying, "Blood is thicker than water." But for a cyclist, blood is thicker without water. Water maintains the smooth-moving volume of your blood, allowing oxygen and nutrients to reach exercising muscles. While riding, we generate tremendous amounts of heat—as much as 15 to 20 times that is produced at rest—and most of this is dissipated by sweating. Because sweat is produced from blood plasma, if you don't drink, blood volume quickly decreases. This starts a vicious cycle in which heart rate increases, performance suffers, sweat rate declines, and body temperature soars. Worst-case scenario? Heat stroke, which can lead to brain damage or death.

Even moderate shortages can affect performance. In one study, seven well-trained men performed three 2-hour cycling trials. They received either no fluid, enough fluid to maintain their body weight (about two standard 22-ounce water bottles per hour), or half that amount. Those deprived of fluids had the worst performance. And performance was better with full fluid replacement than with half replacement. (Now be honest— on how many rides do you drink two bottles per hour?) Even when you're not cycling, inadequate hydration can cause fatigue or headaches.

How Much Is Enough?

It's shamefully simple to get enough fluid, as many studies have confirmed: Drink enough to replace fluid losses. In other words, you should finish a ride weighing the same as you did at the start. (To avoid inaccuracies introduced by sweat-soggy cycling clothes, weighing should be done when you're undressed.) Each pound of weight lost equals two 8-ounce glasses of water, or the better part of a standard water bottle.

On hot, hard rides, sweat rates can reach 2 to 4 pounds per hour, and you simply may not be able to keep up with your losses. But you can limit the extent of dehydration by maximizing stomach emptying and fluid absorption. To do this, drink about two-thirds of a standard bottle immediately before starting your ride. Then drink one-third of a bottle every 10 minutes while in the saddle. (Amounts vary with body size, so experiment.) A high stomach volume helps fluid leave the stomach and enter your bloodstream more quickly.

Another approach to meeting fluid needs on hot rides is to hyperhydrate. Drink one 8-ounce glass of water for each 20 pounds of body weight before riding. (If you weigh 160 pounds, that's eight glasses.) In some studies the water was consumed during a 30-minute span beginning an hour before cycling. In others, it was consumed over 90 minutes beginning 2½ hours beforehand.

Glycerol products, mixed with water, are purported to assist hyperhydration. Although the results aren't completely clear, one study did find improved performance. Some users, however, experienced stomach upset. These products are available at bike shops or other athletic stores.

Caffeine and Energy Drinks

Caffeine is a diuretic. In other words, it increases urination. Some cyclists even believe you'll end up more dehydrated after a cup of coffee than you were before. This isn't true. Caffeine is actually a relatively weak diuretic, and the main reason for that pressing bladder after drinking coffee is that coffee is an excellent source of water. While you won't retain quite as much fluid from a cup of joe as from a glass of water, you will certainly end up more hydrated than you would be with no coffee. It's still a good idea to try to match coffee intake cup for cup with a caffeine-free fluid, but unless you're popping caffeine pills, dehydration isn't a big concern. And many riders like the jolt that a good hit of French roast gives them.

For proper hydration, the most important ingredient in any beverage is water—either straight from the tap or as the major ingredient of a sports drink. Of course, sports drinks have the added advantage of carbohydrate, which provides fuel to your muscles and can improve performance in rides lasting an hour or more. Most sports drinks are 6 to 8 percent carbohydrate—enough to boost performance and still empty from the stomach at a quick-enough rate. In some riders, higher concentrations can slow stomach emptying and may contribute to cramping or nausea. The only way to know how stronger drinks affect you is to experiment.

Postride Replenishment

Despite your best efforts, chances are good that you won't drink enough on the bike to replace 100 percent of the fluid lost on hot days or during hard rides. To make up the deficit, don't stop drinking when you stop pedaling. Here's what you should do as quickly as you can after the ride.

Drink more fluid than you lost. If you finish a ride down 2 pounds, you need to drink more than the equivalent amount of fluid to restore hydration. This is because some fluid inevitably ends up as urine.

Replace electrolytes, primarily sodium. Sodium, either in a drink or solid food, allows the body to retain more fluid. How much sodium should you replace? It's hard to be precise, but including a glass of vegetable juice could help kick-start your rehydration regimen.

Avoid carbonated beverages and alcohol. Drinks like soda and beer aren't the best choice for rehydration. A recent study found that higher levels of carbonation lowered the amount athletes drank after exercise. And alcohol is a diuretic, which can maintain a fluid deficit rather than remedy it.

25
Sports Drinks

Sure, you know that hydrating and refueling are critical to cycling performance. That point has been hammered home since the beginning of this book. But you may need a painful personal experience to really become convinced.

For nutritionist and long-distance cyclist Susan Barr, Ph.D., it happened when she participated in a study that required riding up to 6 hours at a stretch in a heat chamber. For two of the torture sessions, fluid was provided and everyone made it through with stable heart rates and body temperatures. But in the third trial, fluid was withheld. Most subjects didn't make it past 4 hours. One had to quit when his heart rate reached 95 percent of maximum, another when her core temperature hit 104°F (at which risk of heat injury increases). The others succumbed to sheer exhaustion. The experience turned all of them into committed fluid fanatics.

How much liquid you need depends on your personal sweat rate. Get a close approximation by weighing yourself naked before and after riding for a number of days. For example, suppose you drain two standard water bottles during a ride and still lose a couple of pounds. Since one full bottle weighs about 1¼ pounds, you needed to consume two additional bottles to keep up with fluid loss.

Along with fluid, carbohydrate is essential during prolonged exercise. In landmark studies, Edward Coyle, Ph.D., a *Bicycling* magazine Fitness Advisory Board member, showed that elite cyclists who consumed a carbo drink could exercise about an hour longer before exhaustion (4 hours compared to 3) than those who were given only water.

A sports drink can provide the same benefit. As a rule, you should consume 0.33 gram of carbohydrate per pound per hour to prolong performance. So if you weigh 135 pounds, that's 135 × 0.33 = 45 grams per hour. (For a 155-pound rider, it's 52 grams per hour; for a 175-pounder, 58 grams per hour; and for a 195-pounder, 65 grams per hour.) Using a drink that contains the recommended 6 percent carbohydrate, you get 45 grams of carbo in 1⅓ bottles filled with 20 ounces.

How Sports Drinks Compare

DRINK*	PACKAGED AS (20 OZ)	CALORIES (KCAL)	CARBOHYDRATE (MG)	CARBOHYDRATE (%)
Allsport	Liquid	175	50	8.8
Cytomax	Powder	143	30	5.3
Endura	Powder	142	36	6.3
Gatorade	Liquid	125	35	5.9
Powerade	Liquid	175	47.5	8.3
PR Solution	Powder	142	36	6.3
Shaklee Performance	Powder	233	58	10.2
XLR8	Liquid concentrate	138	34.5	6.0

Drinking enough on the bike is a learned skill, so practice drinking frequently even on short rides. When you're out for several hours, begin hydrating and refueling right away. A recent study showed that consuming a large amount of carbohydrate after 2 hours of cycling doesn't maintain performance as well as the same amount taken in smaller doses throughout the first 2 hours.

One other point: One study found that sports drinks are acidic and might lead to tooth decay—particularly because they're consumed over long periods. There's no data on whether this is a special problem for athletes, but until follow-up studies are done, cyclists should be sure to brush their teeth soon after riding and floss regularly. On the bike, consider having water in one bottle to use as a chaser for the sports drink.

Categories

"How Sports Drinks Compare" gives an overview of some sports drinks on the market. Here's a closer look at the information.

Type. Sports drinks come as a powder, liquid, or liquid concentrate. Ready-made liquids are hassle-free, but not as portable as other types.

SODIUM (MG)	SOURCE OF CARBOHYDRATE	VITAMINS AND MINERALS
138	High-fructose corn syrup	B vitamins
150	Starch, maltodextrin	Chromium, vitamin C
107	Fructose, maltodextrin	B vitamins, vitamin C and E, magnesium
275	Sucrose, glucose-fructose	—
137	High-fructose corn syrup, maltodextrin	—
60	Maltodextrin, fructose	B vitamins, vitamin C, chromium
233	Maltodextrin, fructose, glucose	—
111	Glucose, fructose, glucose polymers	—

Powder and liquid concentrate can be carried on long rides and used to make more drink en route. They also let you make a stronger concentration. In general, powders are the least expensive choice.

Calories. Caloric content is listed here in case you're trying to meet (or stay below) a certain amount per day. Keep in mind that total carbohydrate content is what's important for athletic performance.

Carbohydrate grams. Use this figure to calculate how much of the drink you should consume for your body weight, according to the 0.33 gram-per-pound-per-hour formula described above.

Carbohydrate percentage. Drinks should contain about 6 to 8 percent carbohydrate. Substantially less than 6 percent isn't enough to prolong performance; much over 8 percent may cause stomach problems (though individual tolerances vary).

Sodium. Cyclists lose substantial sodium in sweat, but the amount varies with the individual. In general, most riders have enough sodium stored for rides up to 6 hours, and it's easily replaced through food consumption. For longer rides, consider using the higher sodium content of Gatorade and Shaklee Performance. In general, athletes shouldn't be obsessed with avoiding sodium.

Source of carbohydrate. An effective sports drink should provide mainly glucose, the fuel your muscles use. Starch, maltodextrin, glucose polymers, and glucose provide 100 percent glucose, while sucrose and high-fructose corn syrup, often included to improve palatability, provide about 50 percent glucose. Drinks containing mainly fructose may cause digestive problems in some riders because they're absorbed less quickly and pull water into the gastrointestinal tract. You should experiment with these drinks during training to discover any problems.

Vitamins and minerals. There's no need to replace vitamins and trace minerals such as chromium during exercise. Vitamin and mineral deficiencies develop over weeks or months, not during a 4-hour ride.

And what about taste? It's an individual preference. Choose a flavor you can handle even when it becomes warm. After all, if the taste makes it a chore to drink, you probably won't drink enough to get the benefits.

26

Energy Gels

First, there were water and bananas. Next, came sports drinks and energy bars. Now, on-bike nutrition can be found in small packets. Gels, with the consistency of syrup or pudding, contain the carbohydrate you need to survive long rides. The major carbo player may be maltodextrin, rice syrup, or poly/oligosaccharides. In all cases, these break down into glucose, the fuel that your muscles use.

Gels come in single-serving foil packets that are torn open and squeezed or sucked into your mouth. To get the recommended carbohydrate intake (0.6 gram per kilogram of body weight per hour; or 30 to 60 grams each hour for weights from 110 to 220 pounds) you need a gel packet every 30 to 45 minutes. One product, Carb-Boom, is packaged in a plastic cup with a foil lid, containing the equivalent of three servings. For easier use while riding, two Carb-Boom cups can be emptied into a refillable plastic squeeze tube available from the manufacturer.

Do gels work? No doubt. Studies providing wheel-to-wheel comparisons of solid and liquid carbohydrate have yet to be published, however. Research conducted at Ohio State University in Columbus did find that cycling performance was similar when carbohydrate and fluid were combined and consumed in equal amounts either as a sports drink or as an energy bar and water. There's no reason to suspect that an energy gel and water wouldn't produce the same results—as would a bagel and water (or pick your favorite carbohydrate).

You can even make your own gel. Two or three tablespoons of fruit syrup or jelly contain about 25 grams of carbohydrate, providing a similar boost as a gel packet. Look for products that list glucose or sucrose as the first sugar ingredient.

Gels, however, contain more pizzazz than grape jelly. In addition to the electrolytes (sodium and potassium) found in most gels, an array of other ingredients may be mixed in the recipe, including the following:

Medium-chain triglycerides (MCTs). Unlike conventional triglycerides (fats), medium-chain triglycerides don't delay stomach emptying, and research done in the Netherlands has shown that they are used as an energy source during exercise. But because of the relatively small amounts that can be tolerated without unpleasant gastrointestinal symptoms, MCTs provide only 6 or 7 percent of the energy needed during moderate exercise. This is too small to affect carbohydrate use or glycogen breakdown during 3 hours of cycling.

Caffeine/guarana. If you missed your morning coffee, gel with added caffeine or guarana (a Brazilian seed high in caffeine) might give you the lift you need. The amounts added, though, are small—only about 25 mg per gel packet, compared to about 100 mg in a typical cup of coffee. Most studies on the performance-enhancing effects of caffeine have used much higher doses—about 5 mg per kilogram of body weight (300 mg for a 132-pound adult).

Ginseng. In studies at Wayne State University in Detroit, cycling performance was unchanged in men and women who took ginseng for 8 weeks at either the recommended or twice the recommended dose.

Amino acids. It has been suggested that "central fatigue" may contribute to the inability to maintain a given exercise level even when car-

How Energy Gels Compare

GEL	AVG NUTRIENTS PER PACKAGE
Carb-Boom	310 calories; 78 g carbohydrate; 0 g protein; 0 g fat
ClifShot	100 calories; 4 g carbohydrate; 0 g protein; 9 g fat
Extreme Blast	80 calories; 20 g carbohydrate; 0 g protein; 0 g fat
Gatorade ReLode	100 calories; 20 g carbohydrate; 0 g protein; 0 g fat
Gu	100 calories; 20–25 g carbohydrate; 0 g protein; 0–2 g fat
Hammer Gel	100 calories; 24–25 g carbohydrate; 0 g protein; 0–1 g fat
Pocket Rocket	100 calories; 25 g carbohydrate; 0 g protein; 0 g fat
Power Gel	110 calories; 28 g carbohydrate; 0 g protein; 0 g fat
Squeezy	80 calories; 20 g carbohydrate; 0 g protein; 0 g fat
Ultra Gel	133 calories; 24 g carbohydrate; 0 g protein; 4 g fat

bohydrate is provided. In other words, your brain shuts down your legs. The theory is that exercise lowers blood levels of branched-chain amino acids (BCAA) such as valine, leucine, and isoleucine because they are used by working muscles. This leads to an increase in the ratio of tryptophan to the other amino acids with which it competes for transport in the brain. Increased brain tryptophan uptake is thought to lead to increased synthesis of serotonin, a neurotransmitter implicated in fatigue. By taking BCAA during exercise to restore the normal ratio, it is speculated that central fatigue can be avoided.

Does it work? Not according to a study published in the *Journal of Physiology*. Cyclists working at 70 to 75 percent of max VO$_2$ consumed drinks containing carbohydrate and either tryptophan, a low dose of BCAA, or a high dose of BCAA. Despite large differences in blood amino acid levels and estimated brain tryptophan uptake, exercise time to exhaustion didn't differ.

FLAVORS	EXTRAS
Apple-cinnamon	None
Mocha, raspberry, peanut, cocoa peanut, vanilla	Caffeine in two flavors
Cherry cola, coffee, grape, sourberry	Added guarana, ginseng
Banana, grape, unflavored	None
Chocolate, orange, vanilla, berry, banana, plain	Added amino acids; vitamins C and E; herbs including ginseng; caffeine
Chocolate, vanilla, espresso, raspberry, unflavored	Added amino acids
Chocolate, lemon-lime, wild berry, orange	Added chromium, caffeine, and guarana in some flavors
Lemon-lime, strawberry-banana, vanilla, chocolate, tropical fruit	Vitamin C, E; amino acid blend; caffeine, kola nut and ginseng in strawberry-banana and chocolate
Banana, peach, pineapple, lemon-lime, strawberry, vanilla	Added beta-carotene
Banana creme, strawberry creme, unflavored	Fat is medium-chain triglycerides

Chromium. Playing a role in blood glucose regulation, supplemental chromium may help those with impaired glucose tolerance, who are often overweight and inactive. Studies showing an effect on cycling performance have not been done, however.

Decisions, Decisions

So which gel should you choose? No amount of additives or carbohydrates will help if you can't stomach the flavor. Two common complaints about gels are that they're too sweet or have an unpleasant aftertaste.

Cyclists who don't excel at no-hands riding need to use their teeth to open packets. Some are hard to empty completely, leading to a gooey jersey pocket when transporting used packages home. (Obviously they shouldn't be tossed by the road- or trailside. To quote one manufacturer, "Trash the competition, not the planet.")

Gels cost around a dollar a hit, making them an expensive energy source for long rides. If cost is a concern, you might carry a couple of packets for emergency use only and rely on more economical foods and drinks for your routine refueling.

The bottom line: For some cyclists, chewing and swallowing an energy bar while riding is difficult. Others find that a sports drink tastes great in the early hours of a long ride, but 50 miles down the road, they're craving the clean taste of water. For these individuals, gels may be the solution. They don't require chewing and should be chased by water to speed their digestion.

27

The Scoop on Sugar

These days, refined sugar takes the rap for everything from childhood obesity and gaping cavities to the actions of gun-wielding mass murderers. The average American eats 20 teaspoons (320 calories) of refined sugar each day, and that's counting just what's added to our food—not the sugars that occur naturally in fruit, beans, milk, and the like. A cyclist on a 2-hour ride could easily add another 20 teaspoons simply by using recommended amounts of sports drinks, energy bars, or gels.

There are reports of people being addicted or allergic to sugar, and athletes who swear off sugar and begin to perform better. And yet scores of lab studies show that sugar improves endurance on a treadmill or stationary bike, with sugar-laden sports drinks consistently edging out water in head-to-head competitions. So what's the real scoop?

Myth: You can be allergic to sugar.

Fact: It's not possible. Your body needs sugar to survive. Most sugars are eventually converted to glucose, which is absolutely critical for body functioning. It's the primary fuel for your brain and red blood cells as well as for muscle during intense exercise. If your body falls short of glucose, it sacrifices protein to make it.

Myth: Honey is more healthful than refined white sugar.

Fact: Once food is digested and sugars are absorbed, your body can't differentiate the sugar (glucose) it gets from vegetables, fruit, bagels, honey, or a Baby Ruth bar. In whole foods, sugars occur in combination with vitamins, minerals, fiber, protein, fat, and other valuable substances. That's why so-called naturally occurring sugars (those in whole foods) give more nutritional bang for your bagel. Most sugars (including honey, jam, and molasses) contain about 50 calories and 13 grams of carbohydrate per tablespoon, but negligible nutrients.

Myth: Sugar makes you fat.

Fact: The thinking here is that sugar promotes fat gain because it causes an exaggerated insulin response. (Insulin is a hormone that promotes fat storage.) Sugar does lead to insulin release, as does protein, but this is a good thing. The insulin helps glucose and amino acids enter your cells, where glucose is used for fuel and amino acids are used to replace body protein. Most studies show that obesity results far more often from high-fat diets.

Myth: Sugar causes cavities.

Fact: Guilty as charged, and the more time that passes before you brush, the greater the risk. Babies who drink juice from a bottle over a long period are particularly prone, as are cyclists who sip sugary sports drinks for hours at a time.

Myth: Sugar causes disease.

Fact: The Center for Science in the Public Interest, based in Washington, D.C., reported that soft drinks may cause osteoporosis. This is a real concern. In kids who gulp soda instead of milk, bone mass may not increase as much as it should, and the long-term consequence could be an epidemic of osteoporosis. The problem isn't the sugar itself, but that sugary foods tend to displace whole foods such as fruits, vegetables, dairy products, and whole grains—foods that contain fiber, vitamins, minerals, and phytochemicals, all of which protect against disease.

Bottom line: Sugar isn't poison, but its use should be kept in proportion. If you use energy drinks, bars, or gels on rides instead of water and bananas, be sure that the rest of your diet contains lots of whole grains, fruits, and vegetables, but minimal sweets.

28
Cyclists and Calcium

Ask cyclists about their bones, and you'll probably hear tales of cracked clavicles. But there's a lot more to this topic. There are some common myths about an even bigger threat to a cyclist's bones: osteoporosis, the decrease in bone mass and density that can lead to brittleness and frequent fractures. Here's a closer look at these myths along with advice to prevent osteoporosis.

Myth: Being an active cyclist promotes bone health.

Fact: Regular weight-bearing exercise helps build and maintain bone strength. Unfortunately, cycling is not a weight-bearing exercise. The significance of this is clearly demonstrated in a study of Tour de France racers, who often spend as much as 6 hours on the bike, followed by massage and rest. They were discovered to have bone densities that are 8 to 10 percent below that of noncycling adult men of similar age. This finding is backed by several other studies where cyclists' bone densities were lower than that of other athletes or normal active adults.

Myth: Osteoporosis is a women's problem.

Fact: The stereotype of an osteoporosis victim is a fragile, hunched-over, elderly woman. It's true that women are at increased risk, especially after menopause or if their menstrual cycles are disturbed before then. But men get osteoporosis, too. In fact, one-third of all hip fractures occur in men.

Myth: Osteoporosis is an old person's problem.

Fact: Adult bone density, which peaks at age 30, reflects how much was gained during growth, how well it was maintained during early adulthood, and how quickly it is being lost with aging. Heredity plays a big role, so osteoporosis can occur before a person reaches senior-citizen status. But even if you didn't choose your grandparents wisely, there's still a lot you can do right now to build or maintain bone.

Myth: Milk is for kids.

Fact: Calcium is needed in childhood to build a strong skeleton, but it's also required in adulthood to maintain bone health. Milk is a great source. Some people note that in places such as China, people who don't drink milk have few fractures. But physical activity, genetics, the body's geometry, and many dietary components differ between North America and China. In addition, studies within China show higher bone density in people with higher calcium intakes. Milk is beneficial no matter what your age.

Safeguard Your Bones

How can you tell if you're in danger of developing osteoporosis? Risk factors include being female, being underweight, smoking, having a

Where to Find Calcium

FOOD	AMOUNT (OZ)	CALCIUM (MG)
Canned sardines with bones	3	325
Café latte, tall	12	300+
Milk	16	300
Calcium-fortified fruit punch	16	300
Fruit yogurt	6	280
Tofu, made with calcium	8	250
Canned salmon with bones	3	210
Hard cheese (Cheddar, Parmesan)	1	205
Ice cream	8	90
Almonds, roasted	1	80
Cottage cheese	8	80
White beans	8	75
Kale, boiled	8	50
Broccoli, cooked	8	50
Kidney or pinto beans	8	30–40

NOTE: Low-fat or fat-free dairy products contain the same amount of calcium as whole-milk products.

family history of the disease, or being inactive. But the most accurate way to estimate risk is to measure bone density using dual-energy x-ray absorptiometry. The amount of radiation is very low, similar to what you'd get on a cross-country airplane flight. But even if you don't undergo this procedure, it's worth acting on the following nutrition and exercise tips.

Nutrition. Calcium is crucial. You need 1,000 milligrams per day between the ages of 19 and 49, then 1,200 milligrams per day after age 50. (One cup of milk equals 300 milligrams . See "Where to Find Calcium" on page 101 for calcium amounts from other sources.)

Excess protein and sodium cause calcium loss through urination. This is a tough issue for athletes, who need more of both nutrients than sedentary folks. The key is to not overdo protein and sodium intake, and to ensure that generous calcium consumption covers any losses that do occur.

Phosphorus is another nutrient to watch. In an organic form (found in unprocessed foods), it has little effect on calcium. But inorganic forms such as phosphoric acid (sometimes used in cola beverages) may increase urinary calcium loss. So in addition to scoring a zero as sources of calcium, these beverages might eliminate some of the calcium that's already in your body.

Caffeine is another culprit, being associated with poor calcium absorption. But if your calcium intake is within recommended amounts, caffeine's effects are minor. In most cases, it's not the caffeine that causes problems, but the paucity of calcium. So make that next coffee a fat-free latte.

Exercise. All forms of exercise weren't created equal when it comes to benefits to bones. While cycling is great for the cardiovascular system, the forces exerted through pedaling simply aren't enough to stimulate bone growth. No one is suggesting that you hang up your helmet, but you might consider these osteoporosis-fighting strategies.

- Add weight training. Besides helping you become a more powerful cyclist, resistance training increases bone density.

- Add other sports. Bone responds to unusual forces, so try something different. Incorporate weight-bearing cross-training such as running, aerobics, racket sports, basketball, or volleyball. In a British study, simply jumping up and down 50 times a day for 6 months increased young women's hip bone densities by about 4 percent.

■ Take a walk at the end of the day on long rides or bike tours.

29
Alcohol's Effect on Performance

One year, there was a competitor in the Ironman triathlon who rode the cycling leg with a six-pack of beer in his handlebar bag. He claimed that drinking the beer aided his performance. By the end of the 112-mile ride, he had downed all six cans. There's no record of how he did in the ensuing 26-mile run.

If you're like most cyclists, alcohol's role in your riding is probably not quite this overt. You may sip a glass of beer or wine with dinner after a ride, and there's no problem with that. But consider another scenario where you and your riding buddies raise a toast or two (or three or four) to the day's accomplishments. While that's not as extreme as sipping six cold ones in the saddle, drinking that exceeds sensible limits does have a surprisingly large influence on performance.

Drinking's Dangers

When you drink too much, you begin the following day's ride at a disadvantage. In addition to traditional hangover effects such as headache and nausea, you'll probably be dehydrated.

Though it seems contradictory, drinking actually lowers your body's fluid levels. In fact, to metabolize a single ounce of alcohol, your body uses 8 ounces of water. Alcohol, like caffeine, is also a diuretic, which causes increased urination and water loss. Therefore, it's important to replenish any fluid losses before riding. Have one glass of water for every two drinks. (A drink is equal to a 12-ounce beer, a 4-ounce glass of wine, or 1½ ounces of 80-proof liquor. Each of these provides ½ ounce of pure alcohol.)

Even so, don't expect to be at your best. A U.S. Navy study found that it takes 36 hours for your body to fully recover from drunkenness. Interestingly, cycling or other aerobic exercise can speed the recovery by raising your body temperature, thus eliminating the alcohol more quickly.

Nonetheless, too much drinking is still detrimental. On long rides in cold weather, having alcohol in your blood may contribute to hypothermia (dangerously low body temperature). During warm weather, the risk of dehydration, heat exhaustion, and heatstroke increases with the amount of alcohol consumed.

In the broader picture, one-half of all traffic deaths and one-third of all traffic injuries are alcohol-related. It's also a significant factor in home, industrial, and recreational mishaps. And in the long term, excessive alcohol use leads to myriad serious health problems, including liver damage, high blood pressure, and abnormalities of the heart, brain, muscles, and esophagus.

Drinking's Possible Benefits

Despite the dangers of excessive drinking, moderate alcohol consumption has been touted as an effective protector against heart disease because it has been shown to increase the level of HDL (good) cholesterol in the blood. But according to one study, this effect occurs only in sedentary people. As a cyclist, your HDL level is probably already high and your heart is reaping its protective benefits. For you, moderate drinking may provide no added advantage. Similarly, in terms of cycling performance, modest drinking the night before doesn't help. But unlike excessive drinking, it doesn't hurt, either.

Determining the difference between moderate and excessive alcohol intake isn't easy. Some experts say the threshold between harmless and harmful comes after the second drink. Some claim it's okay to have one drink for each 50 pounds of body weight. Others insist that alcohol tolerance depends on the individual.

In any case, you can probably sense when you're reaching your threshold. If you want to ride at 100 percent the following day, it's a good idea to heed your limit.

Alcohol in the Body

To better understand alcohol's effect, you need to understand what happens to it in your system. As you drink, alcohol is absorbed directly from your stomach and small intestine into the bloodstream. This process occurs quickly. (Notice how soon you feel the buzz after starting to drink.) Your body reacts by immediately trying to eliminate the invading alcohol. The liver releases enzymes that begin this breakdown. But your body can get rid of only about ¾ ounce of alcohol per hour (the equivalent of 1½ beers, glasses of wine, or mixed drinks).

Unlike caffeine or other performance enhancers, drinking before or during a ride won't give you an energy boost. Because your liver is busy processing alcohol, it decreases its output of glucose, thus limiting this important muscle fuel and causing premature fatigue during exercise. Meanwhile, the alcohol that is waiting to be processed by the liver is unable to provide any energy for the muscles. Even if it were available, alcohol is a weak energy source because it doesn't contribute to the formation of muscle glycogen, the body's preferred fuel for cycling.

These effects, in addition to dehydration, increase with the amount of alcohol consumed. Naturally, a glass of beer or wine with dinner won't noticeably inhibit your performance, but a few glasses will.

Beer as a Carbo-Loader

Despite the contention of some riders, drinking beer is a poor form of carbo-loading. A 12-ounce beer provides a scant 50 calories of carbohydrate. This isn't much, compared to the effect it has on your central nervous system. For instance, if you weigh 150 pounds, drinking five beers will raise your blood alcohol level to about 0.10, which makes you legally drunk in most states. At the same time, five beers provide only enough carbohydrate to ride about 10 miles.

Wine is an even worse choice. A 4-ounce glass contains just 15 carbohydrate calories. The poorest carbo-loader, however, is liquor, which has no carbohydrate at all.

Alcoholic beverages contain mostly empty calories (they're not accompanied by other nutrients). Beer and wine do provide traces of protein, as well as scant amounts of some vitamins and minerals, but these nutrients are much more abundant in other drinks and foods.

Twelve ounces of regular beer contain about 150 calories. Light beers average around 100. A glass of wine or 1½ ounces of liquor also have about 100 calories. If you're watching your weight, alcohol intake is a good place to look.

30

The Creatine Controversy

Locker-room legend says it will make you bigger, faster, and stronger. Your quads will bulge, you'll fly through sprints, and your weight-training performances will astound your friends. It's cheap and it's widely available.

Is it a steroid, or some exotic and undetectable new drug? No, this miracle supplement is creatine, readily available in health food stores where it sells for as little as 60 cents for 20 grams. It's also legal, not prohibited by the International Olympic Committee or any cycling federation. Once a little-known supplement for power athletes, creatine is now used in many sports, including bike racing.

Naturally, creatine has also prompted research and some concern. At least 17 studies were presented at the 1998 meeting of the American College of Sports Medicine, based in Indianapolis. No one wonders if creatine works—under certain circumstances, it works quite well—but there is concern about whether the supplement could have negative long-term side effects.

What Is It?

Everyone has creatine in their muscles. The body makes it from amino acids (components of protein). It's difficult to boost creatine levels through your diet, however. You would need to eat more than 10 pounds of meat per day to get the same dosage that exists in a single serving of a typical supplement.

What Does It Do?

Your muscles use adenosine triphosphate (ATP) when they contract. For activities lasting more than a few seconds, ATP comes from breaking down carbohydrate and fat. Explosive activities such as sprinting are powered by ATP already in the muscle, which can fuel just a few seconds of all-out exercise. Creatine supplements extend this time by helping to rebuild ATP.

Is It Safe?

Weight lifters and football players have been using creatine for a few years with no evidence of health problems. In 1997, there was speculation that the deaths of three college wrestlers were creatine-related. But these athletes were using dangerous dehydration practices to lose weight, and there's no evidence that creatine contributed to the fatalities. Subjects who used creatine for 28 days showed no harmful effects during blood testing in a 1998 study conducted by Richard Kreider, Ph.D. Anecdotal evidence suggests creatine contributes to muscle cramps and pulls, but this hasn't happened in controlled studies. The most commonly reported side effect is a 1- to 3-pound weight gain. This benefits power athletes, but slows cyclists on climbs if strength gains don't more than compensate for it.

Does It Work?

Creatine can give you a boost on short and repeated bursts such as sprints, intervals, or quick climbs. Some cyclists say that creatine helps them train harder and recover quicker between interval sessions. These benefits remain unproven, however. Others say it helps their endurance, but no research has supported this contention. Interestingly, a Belgian study found that subjects who downed 3 cups of coffee daily derived no benefit from creatine.

31
Cancer-Fighting Foods

Even though heart disease is the primary cause of death for Americans, there's nothing like the thought of cancer to make the blood run cold. It affects us all, young and old—even seemingly superhuman athletes such as Lance Armstrong.

Cancer doesn't follow any rules, but science has shown that it generally follows a few guidelines. Despite its capricious nature, evidence indicates that about one-third of cancer deaths in the United States are related to diet—which puts some control over cancer into your hands. In fact, if you don't smoke, what you eat is your biggest modifiable cancer factor.

Of course, changing your diet won't guarantee that you'll ride into the sunset cancer-free. Genetics are a huge factor. But research indicates that eating right can stack the deck in your favor. Here's how.

Fat

The link between fat and cancer is highly controversial. International comparisons suggest that it is important. For example, fat intake is higher in the United States than in Japan, and the United States has higher rates of certain cancers. But studies don't always find higher cancer rates in those eating more fat. In the Nurses Health Study, the fat intakes of more than 80,000 nurses were assessed over a number of years, and a low-fat diet did not protect them against breast cancer. (The ongoing Women's Health Initiative, in which groups of women will maintain diets of either 20 percent or 30 percent fat for 12 years, should answer this question definitively, but not until 2009.)

What has been confirmed is that too much fat contributes to obesity, and obesity is linked to certain cancers and heart disease. (It will slow you down on hills, too.)

The bottom line: Limit fat to no more than 30 percent of your daily calories and maintain a healthy weight.

Phytoestrogens

Plant hormones, called phytoestrogens, include isoflavonoids (found in soy products) and lignans (found in flaxseed). They've been linked to lower rates of prostate and breast cancer in Asian populations, which eat large amounts of soy. Phytoestrogens also inhibit cancer in cell-culture studies. Research is underway on men who have prostate cancer (or are at high risk) to determine whether soy-supplemented low-fat diets reduce cancer.

Nutrients That Combat Cancer

You know you should avoid alcohol and limit your fat intake. But you can lower your risk for these three common cancers by eating things that have been proven to be effective cancer-fighters.

CANCER	WHAT TO EAT	SOURCES
Prostate	Lycopene	Tomatoes, ketchup
	Antioxidants	Crabs, oysters, vitamin E
	Soy products	Tofu, soy beverages
Breast	Flaxseed	Certain cereals and breads
	Soy products	Tofu, soy beverages
Colon/Rectal	High fiber	Whole grains, beans, legumes, fruits, veggies
	Calcium and vitamin D	Low-fat dairy products

The bottom line: Soy products are a good bet for cancer prevention and may also reduce your risk of heart disease. Buy breads and cereals containing flaxseed, get a vegetarian cookbook, and give those tofu recipes a try.

Heterocyclic Amines

An article in the *Journal of the National Cancer Institute* made the news by reporting that breast cancer risk was 4.62 times greater in women who preferred heavily browned meat than in those who prefer their meat rare or medium. The authors speculate that heterocyclic amines, formed during high-temperature cooking, may be the cause. These compounds cause cancer in animal studies and have been linked to human colon cancer. Unfortunately, the authors only asked the women how they liked their meat cooked, not how much meat they ate, so the results must be interpreted carefully—particularly in light of the food poisoning that can occur from eating undercooked meat.

The bottom line: When cooking meat (unlike when cycling), safety is found in the middle of the road. Cook your meat until it's no longer red, but avoid charring it.

Resveratrol

Found in red wine, resveratrol is a potent antioxidant. Antioxidants inhibit oxidative damage to cells, which is thought to contribute to the risk of cancer and heart disease. In lab studies, resveratrol inhibits all stages of cancer growth in human cancer cells. It also acts biologically against atherosclerosis (hardening of the arteries).

So should you quaff gallons of red wine? It's hard to say. Resveratrol may work when added directly to cells in glass dishes, but whether you absorb useful amounts from wine is open to question. And alcohol in any form has been linked to breast cancer.

The bottom line: Grape juice may be the best dietary source. It provides only half the resveratrol of red wine, but it has no cancer-causing side effects.

Glossary

A

Aerobic: Exercise at an intensity that allows the body's need for oxygen to be continually met. This intensity can be sustained for long periods.

Anaerobic: Exercise above the intensity at which the body's need for oxygen can be met. This intensity can be sustained only briefly.

Anaerobic threshold (AT): *See* Lactate threshold.

B

Blow up: To suddenly be unable to continue at the required pace due to overexertion.

Bonk: A state of severe exhaustion caused mainly by the depletion of glycogen in the muscles because the rider has failed to eat or drink enough. Once it occurs, rest and high-carbohydrate foods are necessary for recovery.

C

Cadence: The number of times during 1 minute that a pedal stroke is completed. Also called pedal rpm.

Carbohydrate: In the diet, it is broken down to glucose, the body's principal energy source, through digestion and metabolism. It is stored as glycogen in the liver and muscles. Carbo can be simple (sugars) or complex (bread, pasta, grains, fruits, vegetables), which contains additional nutrients. One gram of carbohydrate supplies 4 calories.

Cardiovascular: Pertaining to the heart and blood vessels.

Century: A 100-mile ride; a metric century is 100 kilometers (62 miles).

Clydesdale: A heavy rider. At some mountain bike races, there is a Clydesdale class for riders who weigh more than 200 pounds.

Contact patch: The portion of a tire in touch with the ground.

Criterium: A mass-start race covering numerous laps of a course that is normally 1 mile or less in length.

Cross-training: Combining sports for mental refreshment and physical conditioning, especially during cycling's off-season.

D

Drafting: Riding closely behind another rider to take advantage of the windbreak (slipstream), which uses about 20 percent less energy. Also called sitting in or wheelsucking.

E

Electrolytes: Substances such as sodium, potassium, and chloride that are necessary for muscle contraction and maintenance of fluid levels.

F

Fat: In the diet, it is the most concentrated source of food energy, supplying 9 calories per gram. Stored fat provides about half the energy required for low-intensity exercise.

Feed zone: A designated area on a race course where riders can be handed food and drinks.

G

Gastric: Pertaining to the stomach.

Glucose: A sugar, glucose is used for energy by muscles and is the only fuel that can be used by the brain and nervous system. Also called blood glucose.

Glycogen: A fuel derived as glucose (sugar) from carbohydrate and stored in the muscles and liver. It's the primary energy source for high-intensity cycling. Reserves are normally depleted after about 2½ hours of riding.

Glycogen window: The period within an hour after exercise when depleted muscles are most receptive to restoring their glycogen content. By eating foods or drinking fluids rich in carbohydrate, energy stores and recovery are enhanced.

Gorp: Good ol' raisins and peanuts, a high-energy mix for nibbling during rides. Can also include nuts, seeds, M&Ms, or granola.

H

Hamstrings: The muscles on the backs of the thighs; not well-developed by cycling.

I

Intervals: A structured method of training that alternates brief, hard efforts with short periods of easier riding for partial recovery.

L

Lactate threshold (LT): The exertion level beyond which the body can no longer produce energy aerobically, resulting in the buildup of lactic acid. This is marked by muscle fatigue, pain, and shallow, rapid breathing. Also called anaerobic threshold (AT).

Lactic acid: A substance formed during anaerobic metabolism when there is incomplete breakdown of glucose. It rapidly produces muscle fatigue and pain. Also called lactate.

M

Max VO$_2$: The maximum amount of oxygen that can be consumed during all-out exertion. This is a key indicator of a person's potential in cycling and other aerobic sports. It's largely genetically determined but can be improved somewhat by training.

O

Overtraining: Deep-seated fatigue, both physical and mental, caused by training at an intensity or volume too great for adaptation.

Oxygen debt: The amount of oxygen that must be consumed to pay back the deficit incurred by anaerobic work.

P

Paceline: A group formation in which each rider takes a turn breaking the wind at the front before pulling off, dropping to the rear position, and riding the others' draft until at the front once again.

Power: The combination of speed and strength.

Protein: In the diet, it is required for tissue growth and repair. Composed of structural units called amino acids, protein is not a significant energy source unless not enough calories and carbohydrate are consumed. One gram of protein equals 4 calories.

Pull, pull through: Take a turn at the front of the paceline.

Q

Quadriceps: The large muscle in front of the thigh, the strength of which helps determine a cyclist's ability to pedal with power. "Quads" for short.

R

RDA: Abbreviation for Recommended Dietary Allowance, the amount of a given nutrient that should be consumed during a day.

RPM: Abbreviation for "revolutions per minute."

S

Sitting in: *See* Drafting.

Speed: The ability to accelerate quickly and maintain a very fast cadence for brief periods.

T

Training glycogen depletion: A condition caused by several successive days of low carbohydrate intake; characterized by fatigue and lackluster performance.

Index

Underscored page references indicate boxed text.